Understanding Alzheimer's Disease

Andrea C. Nakaya

ReferencePoint Press

San Diego, CA

ReferencePoint Press®

For more information, contact:
ReferencePoint Press, Inc.
PO Box 27779
San Diego, CA 92198
www.ReferencePointPress.com

LIBRARY OF CONGRESS CATALOGING-IN-PUBLICATION DATA

Name: Nakaya, Andrea C., 1976- author
Title: Understanding Alzheimer's Disease/by Andrea C. Nakaya.
Description: San Diego, CA : ReferencePoint Press, Inc, [2027] | Includes bibliographical references and index.
Identifiers: LCCN 2026000021 (print) | LCCN 2026000022 (ebook) | ISBN 9781678213749 library binding | ISBN 9781678213756 ebook
Subjects: LCSH: Alzheimer's disease--Juvenile literature
Classification: LCC RC523.3 .N35 2027 (print) | LCC RC523.3 (ebook)
LC record available at https://lccn.loc.gov/2026000021
LC ebook record available at https://lccn.loc.gov/2026000022

Contents

A Frighteningly Common Disease

Alzheimer's is a brain disease that gets progressively worse over time and for which there is no cure. Many people find it terrifying, and for good reason. The disease usually starts by affecting memory and cognition, and people have trouble remembering information or events or completing familiar tasks. Eventually, they are unable to recognize even close family members, have trouble talking, and can no longer perform everyday tasks like dressing or feeding themselves. As Alzheimer's worsens and affects more of a person's brain, many end up bedridden and struggle even to swallow food and water. This disease is fatal and very common. According to the National Institutes of Health, it is the seventh-leading cause of death in the United States.

A Life-Altering Disease

Alzheimer's is life-altering for those who have it and gradually lose both their mental and physical abilities, as well as for their friends and family members, who helplessly watch this loss happen. Aidan Christy talks about how Alzheimer's affected his grandmother over the last thirteen years of her life. He says:

> My family and I saw my grandma's mind deteriorate slowly, but gradually. It was a very traumatic process. We watched helplessly as her brain slowly began to forget us. Slowly she lost the sense of her personality and her person. That to me is the scariest part of dementia, just knowing you can't do anything to prevent your mind

from slowly wiping away every memory and every person you've ever known. Eventually, my grandmother forgot how to perform daily tasks that we all have to do, such as chewing and eating food or how to drink properly. Her Alzheimer's was getting worse and worse. Seeing her the day before she passed was the most traumatic thing I've gone through, even to this day. I still think about her and her condition too much.[1]

Embracing Small Victories

> "My family and I saw my grandma's mind deteriorate slowly, but gradually. It was a very traumatic process."[1]
>
> —Aidan Christy, grandson to a woman with Alzheimer's

As frightening as Alzheimer's is, people throughout the United States and all over the world have no choice but to live with it every day. Most say that this disease is one of the biggest challenges they have ever had to face and have heartbreaking stories to prove it. However, some people also say that as they or their loved ones fight Alzheimer's, there are occasional bright spots in the darkness. For instance, some say that they learn more about themselves and each other, can still find ways to connect, and feel like the love they have for one another does not go away, despite the many ways their lives change.

Owen Darnell's grandmother developed Alzheimer's when Darnell was a child, fighting it for eight years before she passed away at age seventy-two. Darnell explains that while it was a heartbreaking experience, there were "small victories" that her family enjoyed. She says:

Despite how cruel this disease can be, I was always able to experience glimmers of hope and joy. Sometimes, Grandma would have moments of clarity. We'd see glimpses of her personality during our visits to the memory unit. Despite the hardship, it brought us so much joy to witness those brief moments of familiarity: a mischievous smile and a wink while she pocketed cherry tomatoes from the garden; a warm smile stretching across her face while going through photo albums. . . . Frustration, self-pity, and grief are normal reactions, but there is a way to leave those emotions at bay and treasure the happy moments amidst all the pain.[2]

Joining the Fight

While stories about Alzheimer's are often painful to hear, this disease is so prevalent that it is highly likely that most people will eventually be affected by it in some way. According to the Alzheimer's San Diego organization, every sixty-seven seconds someone in the United States develops Alzheimer's disease. The Alzheimer's Association reports that approximately one in nine Americans over age sixty-five have Alzheimer's, which adds up to more than 7 million people. As these statistics show, this

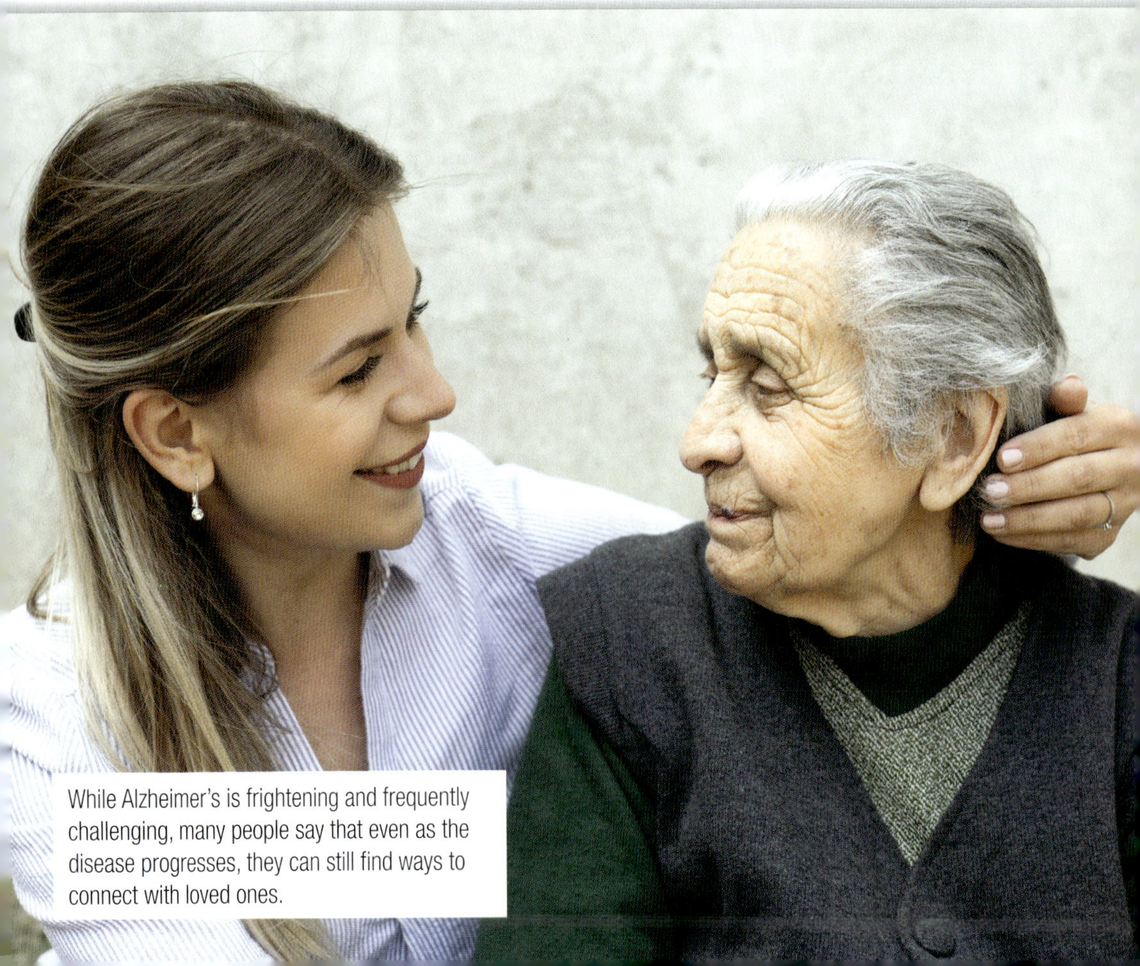

While Alzheimer's is frightening and frequently challenging, many people say that even as the disease progresses, they can still find ways to connect with loved ones.

disease is frighteningly common; so common that most people will eventually either experience it themselves or watch somebody they know struggle with it.

Rather than ignoring this often-uncomfortable topic, some people choose to become better educated about it. Learning more can help reduce the misunderstanding and stigma associated with Alzheimer's so that the people who have it receive better treatment. It can also help people be more prepared for the challenges associated with this disease if they or a friend or family member one day find themselves fighting it. Bart Brammer lives with Alzheimer's. "Don't be ignorant or in denial about the disease," he insists. "Get educated about it. Some people might be afraid to learn what it really is or feel uncomfortable talking about it, but we need everyone in order to fight this."[3]

> "Frustration, self-pity, and grief are normal reactions, but there is a way to leave those emotions at bay and treasure the happy moments amidst all the pain."[2]
>
> —Owen Darnell, granddaughter to a woman with Alzheimer's

Chapter One

What Is Alzheimer's Disease?

Alzheimer's is a type of brain disease. The human brain only weighs about 3 pounds (1.4 kg), but it is an incredible organ that is more powerful than a computer. It is made up of billions of neurons, or nerve cells, which communicate with one another through chemical and electrical signals that pass across the synapses, or spaces between them. Different areas, or lobes, of the brain control different types of functions such as memory, movement, and speech. Overall, the brain controls everything a person thinks and does, and it stores all their memories. However, because the brain controls so much of what happens in the body, when something goes wrong—as happens with Alzheimer's—there are significant problems.

Brain Changes and Dementia

When a person gets Alzheimer's, the neurons and synapses in their brain deteriorate, which stops the brain from doing its job properly. This disease is incurable and is progressive, meaning that it gets worse over time. For most people with Alzheimer's, the part of the brain that controls memory, thinking, and language is affected first, and as a result, they might have trouble remembering things, solving problems, and finding the right words to express their thoughts. As other parts of the brain are affected, they might experience mood changes, have trouble with balance or fine motor skills like writing, and have difficulty communicating. Eventually, they may not recognize friends or family members or know where they are. In advanced stages, patients might have difficulty moving or even swallowing.

When people talk about Alzheimer's, they frequently use the term *dementia*. This word is used to describe the decline in cognitive abilities like remembering, reasoning, and problem-solving that happens with this disease. Alzheimer's is a type of dementia, and it is the most common type, accounting for 60 to 80 percent of all cases, according to the Alzheimer's Association. However, there are other types of dementia that are not Alzheimer's, including vascular dementia, Lewy body dementia, and frontotemporal dementia. These other types of dementia have different causes compared to Alzheimer's and may include other types of symptoms. For instance, vascular dementia is caused by reduced blood flow to the brain, and its early symptoms often include trouble with walking and balance in addition to cognitive problems.

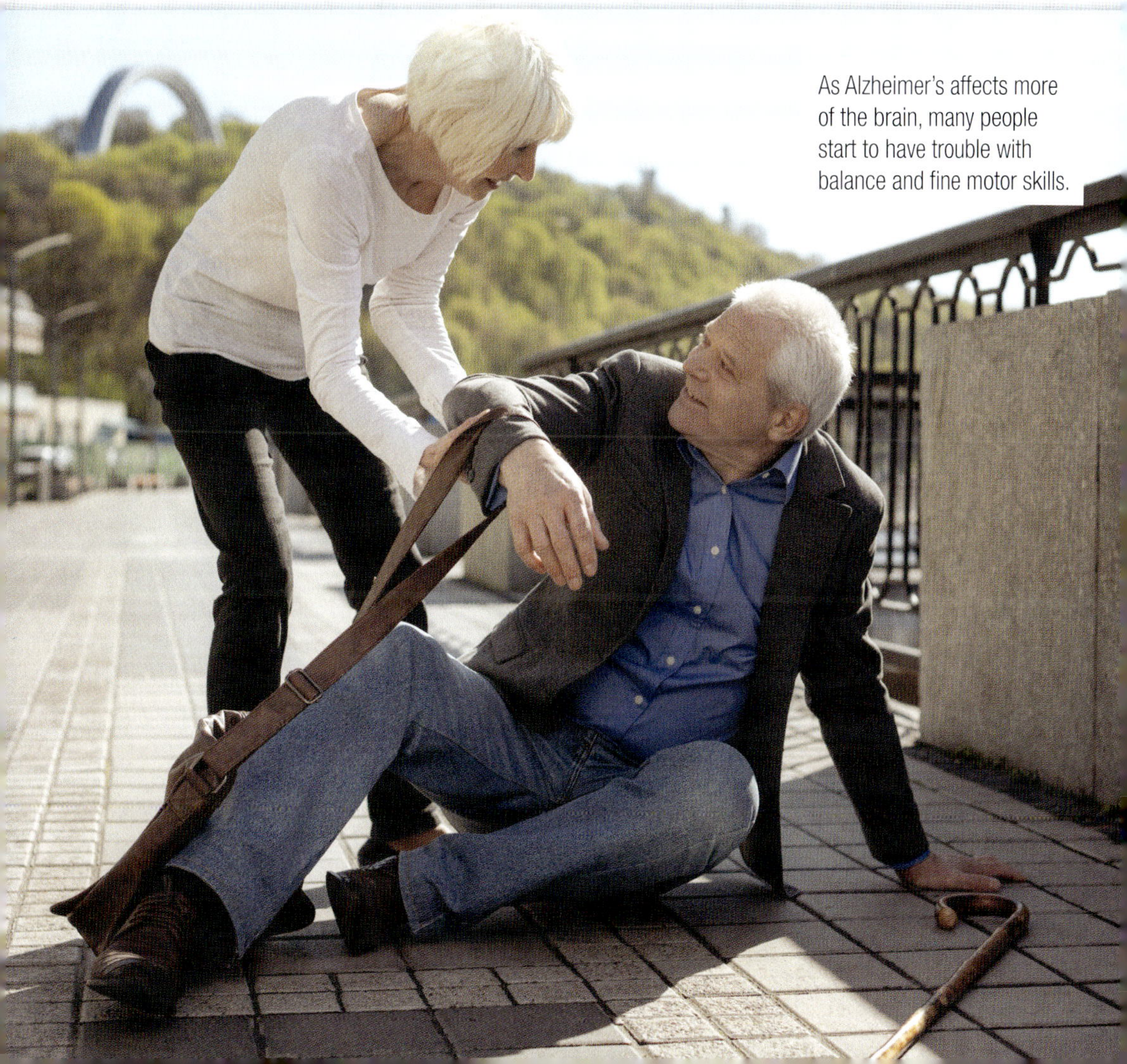

As Alzheimer's affects more of the brain, many people start to have trouble with balance and fine motor skills.

Alzheimer's vs. Senior Moments

Forgetfulness is one of the first symptoms of Alzheimer's and one of the most well-known, but it is important to understand that the forgetfulness that comes with this disease is not the same as the forgetfulness associated with older age. As people age, moments of forgetfulness often become more frequent and more severe. In fact, the forgetfulness associated with old age is so common that the term *senior moment* has been coined to describe it. A recent Reddit text thread asked readers to share their worst senior moment. One person said, "Last month I drove to a granddaughter's house for dinner. She and her husband were very happy to see me. It was the wrong granddaughter's house." Another person said, "I drove off [from the grocery store] with my bags still in the cart. Got home . . . oh crap . . . drove back and there they were."[4]

While these momentary lapses may be annoying or embarrassing, they are generally considered to be a normal part of aging. The forgetfulness associated with Alzheimer's is something different. It is not normal, and it significantly disrupts a person's daily life. Hailey Corum is a teen who lives in San Diego. Her grandfather has Alzheimer's and had to move in with Corum's family because his forgetfulness was impeding his ability to properly care for himself. Some days, she says, her grandfather cannot remember who he is or what year it is, and he has almost burned the house down mul-

Alzheimer's and Sleep Problems

People who have Alzheimer's often experience sleep problems, such as waking up more frequently at night and falling asleep during the day. According to the Mayo Clinic, "Sleep troubles may affect up to 25% of people with mild to moderate Alzheimer's and about 50% of people with moderate to severe Alzheimer's. Sleep troubles tend to get worse as Alzheimer's becomes worse." In addition, some people with Alzheimer's experience something called "sundowning," where they feel more confused and agitated in the late afternoon and in the night. This also makes it more difficult to sleep. Not sleeping well can make symptoms like confusion, memory problems, or agitation worse, so treatment for Alzheimer's often includes strategies for improving sleep.

Mayo Clinic, "Alzheimer's: Managing Sleep Problems," October 30, 2024. www.mayoclinic.org.

tiple times by forgetting to turn the kitchen stove off. In addition, "he forgets people's names, so he just calls everyone 'hey you.'" One day, she says, "my grandpa forgot who my mom was, thinking he lives with his daughters from another marriage and that I was his daughter."[5]

Alzheimer's and Age

While the forgetfulness that comes with Alzheimer's is not a normal part of aging, this is still primarily a disease that occurs in the elderly. In most cases it develops sometime after age sixty-five. Furthermore, the Alzheimer's Association explains that the older a person gets, the more likely they are to develop this disease. "The percentage of people with Alzheimer's dementia increases dramatically with age. Five percent of people age 65 to 74, 13.2% of people age 75 to 84, and 33.4% of people age 85 or older have Alzheimer's dementia," the association says. However, it notes that while a person's risk of Alzheimer's increases with age, the disease is not something that automatically comes with older age. The organization stresses, "It is important to note that Alzheimer's dementia is not a normal part of aging, and older age alone is not sufficient to cause Alzheimer's dementia."[6]

> "The percentage of people with Alzheimer's dementia increases dramatically with age."[6]
>
> —Alzheimer's Association

More rarely, Alzheimer's affects younger people who are only in their thirties, forties, or fifties; in this case it is known as early-onset Alzheimer's. This form of the disease is often aggressive, with symptoms progressing more quickly than in older people who have the disease. There are not a lot of official statistics on this type of Alzheimer's, but according to the Alzheimer's Association, approximately two hundred thousand Americans have early-onset dementia, a number that includes Alzheimer's.

Because most people see Alzheimer's as an older person's disease, a diagnosis of early-onset Alzheimer's can be extremely difficult to deal with. Anitra Mostacero was diagnosed with early-onset Alzheimer's when she was in her forties. She says that she started to realize that something was wrong when she was sitting

"The first year of my diagnosis, I went through a heavy depression, very much mourning the future I felt was ruined."[7]

—Anitra Mostacero, diagnosed with early-onset Alzheimer's

in her car one day and could not remember how to turn it on. She says, "I remember being very confused and thinking, 'what am I doing here? How do I do it?'" She explains that after being diagnosed, she was told she would only have about five to eight good years before she would start to decline cognitively. It was then that she realized the severity of her disease. She says, "The first year of my diagnosis, I went through a heavy depression, very much mourning the future I felt was ruined."[7]

Early Symptoms of Alzheimer's

Every person experiences Alzheimer's differently. However, for most, the early symptoms are relatively mild and not severe enough to stop them from living a fairly a normal life. For many people, one of the first symptoms of this disease is changes in memory. They might have trouble remembering what they did or said recently. They might lose

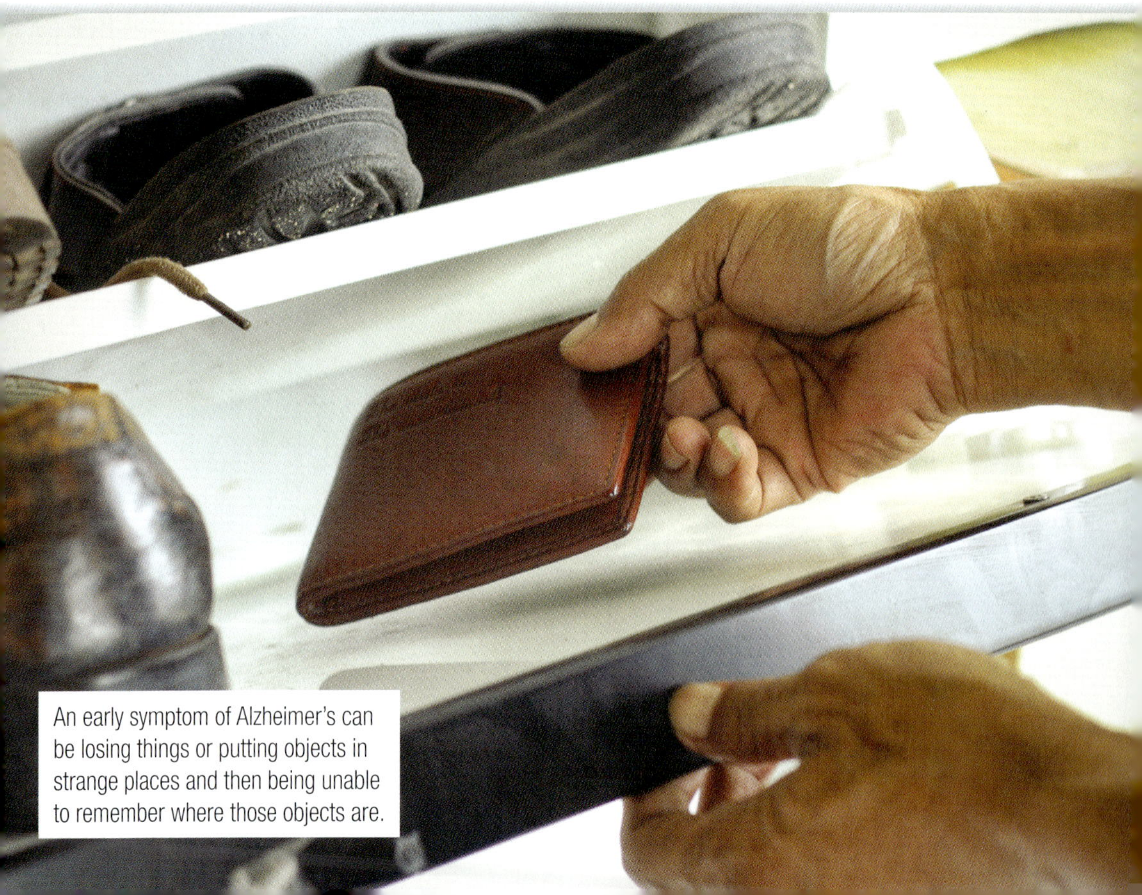

An early symptom of Alzheimer's can be losing things or putting objects in strange places and then being unable to remember where those objects are.

The Economic Cost of Alzheimer's

Caring for people who have Alzheimer's is expensive. On top of medical tests and medication costs, there is the expense of caregiving, with full-time care being needed as the disease becomes more severe. Altogether, this adds up to billions of dollars every year in the United States alone. According to the Alzheimer's Impact Movement, "Alzheimer's is one of the most expensive diseases in America." The organization says more is spent on Alzheimer's than cancer or heart disease, reporting, "In the last five years of life, the costs of a person with dementia, on average, total more than $287,000 (in 2010 dollars). This is compared with $175,000 for a person with heart disease, and $173,000 for someone with cancer." Overall, the organization finds that the United States spends about $360 billion per year caring for people who have Alzheimer's and other dementias.

Alzheimer's Impact Movement, "Fact Sheet: Costs of Alzheimer's to Medicare and Medicaid," 2024. https://alzimpact.org.

things, ask the same questions multiple times, forget the names of objects or people, or forget how to complete tasks that have always been easy. Another common early symptom is trouble with thinking and problem-solving. For instance, a person might have trouble managing their money or making decisions. Mike Balson and his wife Julia talk about Mike's early symptoms. Julia says, "I found a paycheck in a cookbook." Mike says, "I kept asking for directions to go to work, and it once took 20 minutes to do a bank deposit which was unusual because I always had a keen mind."[8]

In the early stages of Alzheimer's, most people understand that their brain is not working as it should, but they feel powerless to do anything about it. Emily Clionsky and Mitchell Clionsky, authors of *Dementia Prevention: Using Your Head to Save Your Brain*, talk about memory problems specifically and explain how frustrating it can feel to be unable to do anything about them. "It is like holding a fistful of sand in your hand—no matter how tightly you squeeze your fingers, the sand slips and slides out, leaving you nearly empty-handed."[9]

Alzheimer's Progression

As the disease progresses, it is common to have both good and bad days. Generally, however, the symptoms become more severe over time, with people becoming more forgetful and confused.

Jonathan Graff-Radford and Angela M. Lunde, Alzheimer's experts and authors of *Mayo Clinic on Alzheimer's Disease and Other Dementias*, explain, "At this stage, it's not uncommon for a person to forget the day of the week or lose track of the season. The person may confuse family members or close friends with one another, or mistake strangers for family."[10] Other symptoms include speech problems and feelings of anxiety or agitation. Alzheimer's can also cause personality changes, such as becoming withdrawn or depressed or being irritable or aggressive. Alzheimer's patients may also behave inappropriately, such as making racist or sexually inappropriate comments.

As the disease becomes even more severe, many people are unable to perform basic daily activities such as washing and feeding themselves or using the bathroom. Eventually, most need full-time help. Some people also become restless or easily upset, imagine things that are not there, or lash out physically.

Wandering is another common symptom of Alzheimer's. A person may simply walk away from their home, and because of their cognitive and memory problems they get lost and cannot find their way back. The Alzheimer's Association reports that six out of ten people with dementia wander at least once, and a significant number wander often. Wandering can be dangerous and result in injury or even death. For instance, the person could fall or get hit by a car.

Laury, who lives in the United Kingdom, observed many of these symptoms with her mother Jacquelyn as her mother's Alzheimer's became more severe. Laury describes their experiences:

> She had become increasingly impaired to the point it was no longer safe for her to live at home. She had forgotten how to use the shower. Her oven had dust on it—she had forgotten how to use it, and most often would forget to eat. . . . She would walk about constantly and then get lost. She took to withdrawing thousands of pounds from her bank account with her pin number written on the back

> of the card. I would finish work and have fifteen missed calls from her neighbours telling me that she, again, had been brought home by a member of the public, completely disorientated.[11]

Laury says that eventually, her mother forgot how to walk or even eat. She explains:

> It was not just a case of forgetting what certain foods were for. She could no longer work out how to eat, having no concept of what a knife or fork was even for. Her word-finding ability became non-existent. Words failed her. She no longer knew how to talk, and communication became more and more difficult. Eventually, as her body finally failed her, she became bed-bound, and I witnessed Alzheimer's parting shot. She lost the ability to swallow. And when you can't swallow, you can't eat.[12]

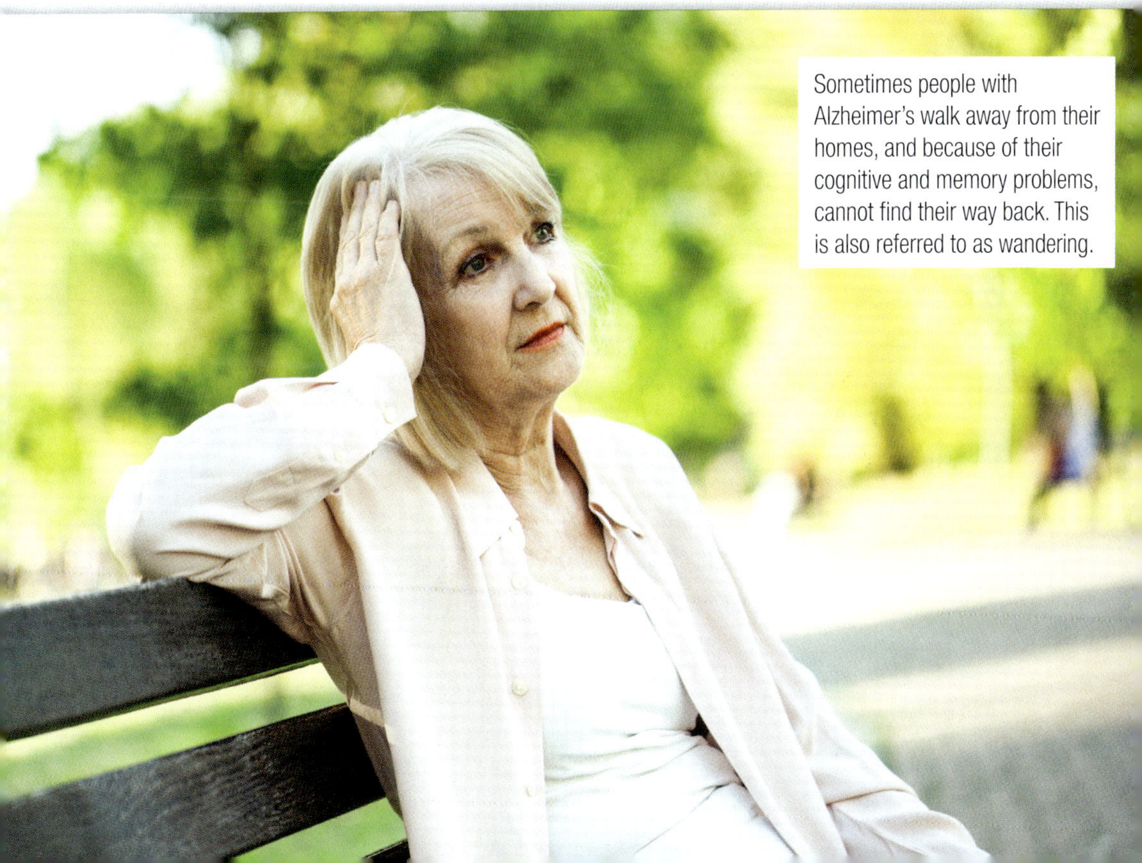

Sometimes people with Alzheimer's walk away from their homes, and because of their cognitive and memory problems, cannot find their way back. This is also referred to as wandering.

A Common Cause of Death

Alzheimer's is incurable and gets progressively worse; eventually the patient dies. According to the Centers for Disease Control and Prevention (CDC), Alzheimer's is the seventh-leading cause of death for adults in the United States. The agency adds, "The actual number of older people who die from Alzheimer's may be much higher than what is officially recorded. Alzheimer's and other types of dementia are not always reported on death certificates."[13] Alzheimer's is not just a problem in the United States; it is also a significant cause of death worldwide.

"The actual number of older people who die from Alzheimer's may be much higher than what is officially recorded. Alzheimer's and other types of dementia are not always reported on death certificates."[13]

—Centers for Disease Control and Prevention

People who die from Alzheimer's typically do so due to complications related to the disease. The most common complication is aspiration pneumonia. As Alzheimer's becomes more advanced, people start to have trouble swallowing and can accidentally inhale food or liquids into their lungs. The bacteria in the food or liquid grow inside the lungs, and the patient develops pneumonia, which can be fatal. Other complications that can be fatal include severe malnutrition (also due to trouble swallowing) and blood clots or serious falls that are consequences of mobility problems.

Overall, Alzheimer's is a serious disease, which has a major impact on society, with billions of dollars spent on health care and long-term care and a significant loss of productivity and quality of life for those affected. Many experts predict that this impact is likely to worsen in the future. For instance, the Alzheimer's Association predicts that unless there is a medical breakthrough in treatment soon, by 2050, 12.7 million Americans over age sixty-five will be living with Alzheimer's disease.

Chapter Two

Why People Get Alzheimer's Disease

Andrea Kline is seventy-one years old and says that her mother, her mother's sister, and her uncle all had Alzheimer's disease. Kline says she is terrified that she will develop it too. She says, "I worry about dementia incessantly. Every little thing that goes wrong, I'm convinced it's the beginning."[14] Kline is not alone in her fears. Surveys consistently shows that Alzheimer's is one of the most feared diseases among older adults. In the United States alone, billions of dollars are spent on research every year to better understand what causes this disease, so that people like Kline will not feel so helpless in facing it. This research has resulted in a better understanding of what Alzheimer's does in the body and the development of more effective drugs to slow its progression. However, scientists have still not found the answer to the question of what causes it in the first place.

Changes in the Brain

While the cause of Alzheimer's remains unknown, researchers do know that people who have Alzheimer's experience specific types of brain changes. This understanding dates back more than a hundred years to German psychiatrist Alois Alzheimer, who first described these changes. In 1901 Alzheimer began treating a woman named Auguste Deter, who was experiencing memory loss, confusion, language problems, and changes in behavior. Her condition deteriorated rapidly, and after she died in 1906, Alzheimer examined her brain. He found that her brain did not look like a typical brain for a person her age; instead, he saw many of the changes that are now known to be signs of

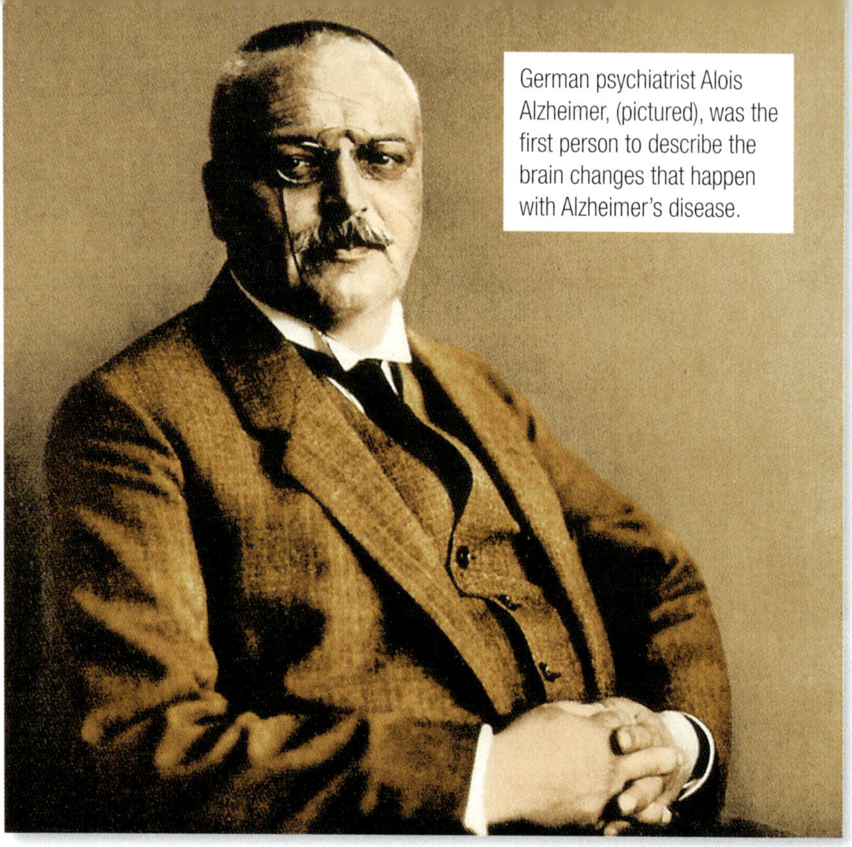

German psychiatrist Alois Alzheimer, (pictured), was the first person to describe the brain changes that happen with Alzheimer's disease.

Alzheimer's disease. Alzheimer published a paper describing his observations, and many people believe this to be the first clinical description of the disease. In recognition of his discovery, Alzheimer's disease was named after him in 1910, when it was included in the eighth edition of a German handbook for psychiatry.

Amyloid Plaques and Tau Tangles

One type of brain change associated with Alzheimer's is that protein clumps known as beta-amyloid plaques start to form in the areas around brain cells, or neurons. Mayo Clinic authors Jonathan Graff-Radford and Angela M. Lunde explain that everyone has beta-amyloid in their body, but in people with Alzheimer's, too much of it accumulates. They say, "In Alzheimer's disease, either too much beta-amyloid is produced or not enough of it is removed during the brain's nightly cleansing process to get rid of waste products."[15] As a result, this substance accumulates into clumps and hardens into what are known as plaques. These plaques stop a person's neurons from functioning correctly.

Another type of protein buildup that happens with Alzheimer's is something called tau tangles. Like beta-amyloid, tau also occurs normally in the human body; it serves important purposes, including helping deliver nutrients to brain cells. However, in Alzheimer's disease, tau strands start unraveling and clumping together. Like beta-amyloid, tau tangles make it more difficult for the brain to work properly. Graff-Radford and Lunde state, "The tangles . . . disrupt its transport system, preventing nutrients and messages from getting to where they're needed. This leads to a breakdown in how well brain neurons are able to function."[16]

Gradual Deterioration

As beta-amyloid and tau tangles accumulate, a person's neurons stop working as they should, and the connections between them break down. Neurons start to die, and the brain begins to shrink as a result. When researchers use brain scans to compare the brain of an Alzheimer's patient with that of a healthy person, they see that it has fewer brain cells and connections and is significantly smaller overall. This deterioration affects almost everything

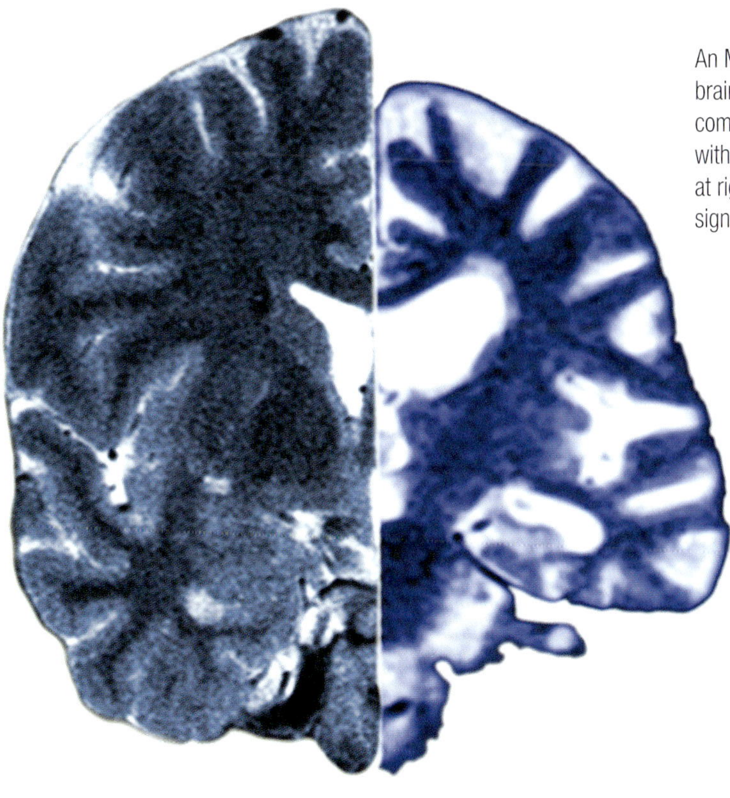

An MRI of a normal brain, at left, compared to a brain with Alzheimer's, at right, which is significantly smaller.

Biomarkers

Medical experts often use the term *biomarker* in relation to diagnosing Alzheimer's disease. Biomarkers—or biological markers—are measurable biological changes that happen in the body as a result of Alzheimer's. Doctors keep track of them as one way to understand whether a person has this disease and how it is progressing. A protein called beta-amyloid is one biomarker, and doctors measure it through brain imaging or by analyzing spinal fluid. Some Alzheimer's researchers focus their work on trying to gain a better understanding of the biomarkers associated with this disease and developing easier ways to test for them. Doing so will improve both diagnosis and treatment in the future.

that happens in the brain, including thinking, remembering, and motor functions like walking and talking.

Most patients are diagnosed with Alzheimer's after they have begun to experience symptoms of the disease. However, scientists have discovered that the changes in the brain that happen with Alzheimer's usually start years before any symptoms appear. This is referred to as the preclinical stage of Alzheimer's disease. In the preclinical stage, a person does not know that anything is wrong, but their brain is already changing, with amyloid plaques and tau tangles forming and neurons starting to deteriorate and lose their connections with other neurons. Researchers think the preclinical stage can last anywhere from ten to twenty-five years.

Risk Factors

While researchers know that brain changes occur in every person who has Alzheimer's, they do not fully understand why these many changes happen. Most believe that there is not one single cause of Alzheimer's, but that this disease is likely caused by a combination of genetic, environmental, and lifestyle factors.

There is strong evidence that specific genetic variations make Alzheimer's disease more likely or unlikely. Every person has their own unique genetic makeup, and these unique variations play a role in the way that their body functions, including diseases that they get. Researchers have identified more than seventy genetic variations that are believed to play a part in the development of Alzheimer's. For example, there is a gene called the apolipoprotein E gene. If a person has one specific type of variation of this gene, they have a higher risk of developing Alzheimer's, while if they have another type of variation, they are less likely to develop it. However, researchers caution that while genetics seems to play a role in this disease, genes alone do not determine whether a person gets Alzheimer's. For instance, some people with a family history of the disease do not develop it, and others with no family history do develop it. The National Institute on Aging explains that genes likely work in combination with many other factors. "In most cases, Alzheimer's does not have a single genetic cause. Instead, it can be influenced by multiple genes in combination with lifestyle and environmental factors,"[17] says the institute.

> "In most cases, Alzheimer's does not have a single genetic cause. Instead, it can be influenced by multiple genes in combination with lifestyle and environmental factors."[17]
>
> —National Institute on Aging

Sex and Ethnicity

In addition to being more likely with specific genetic variations, Alzheimer's is more likely to occur in women and more prevalent in certain ethnic groups. According to the Alzheimer's Association, in the United States two-thirds of the people who live with Alzheimer's are women. Researchers do not completely understand why this is the case. One long-held theory is that because women live longer than men on average, women have a greater likelihood of developing Alzheimer's. In recent years, some researchers have also theorized that there may be some kind of connection between the hormonal changes that women experience in menopause and the development of this disease.

Alzheimer's disease is also more common in Hispanic and Black adults. Specifically, the Alzheimer's Association reports that in the United States, Black adults are approximately twice as likely to have it as White adults, and Hispanic adults are about one and a half times more likely to have it than White adults. As with sex differences, the reasons behind ethnic differences are not well understood.

Health Conditions

Several health conditions are also associated with a higher likelihood of developing Alzheimer's disease. People with cardiovascular disease are more likely to develop Alzheimer's. The cardiovascular system is made up of the heart, blood, and blood vessels, and one of its jobs is to take oxygen- and nutrient-rich blood to the brain and take away waste products. When a person has cardiovascular disease, the heart and blood vessels do not do this work as well, which researchers think may increase the risk of developing Alzheimer's. Unmanaged high blood pressure also affects the ability of the brain to receive oxygen and nutrients and get rid of waste and is likewise thought to increase the risk of Alzheimer's.

Another risk factor for Alzheimer's is diabetes. A number of studies have shown that people who have diabetes have a higher chance of developing Alzheimer's as well. Diabetes is a medical condition in which a person's body does not produce enough insulin or respond to insulin as it should, resulting in high blood sugar levels. Researchers think that the chemical changes that happen in the brain as a consequence of diabetes can contribute to the buildup of beta-amyloid and tau.

Certain types of injury are also known to increase the risk of Alzheimer's. One is hearing loss. Researchers do not have a good understanding of why, but they have found that people

Deterministic Genes

The are certain genes—known as risk genes—that increase a person's risk of developing Alzheimer's disease but do not guarantee it. A very small number of people, however, are born with deterministic genes, which mean that they will almost definitely get Alzheimer's. The Alzheimer's Association explains, "Deterministic genes directly cause a disease, virtually guaranteeing that anyone who inherits one will develop a disorder. Scientists have found rare genes that cause Alzheimer's in only a few hundred extended families worldwide." The organization explains that these deterministic genes cause an early-onset form of Alzheimer's, although such genes are very rare, accounting for less than 1 percent of all cases.

Alzheimer's Association, "Is Alzheimer's Genetic?," 2025. www.alz.org.

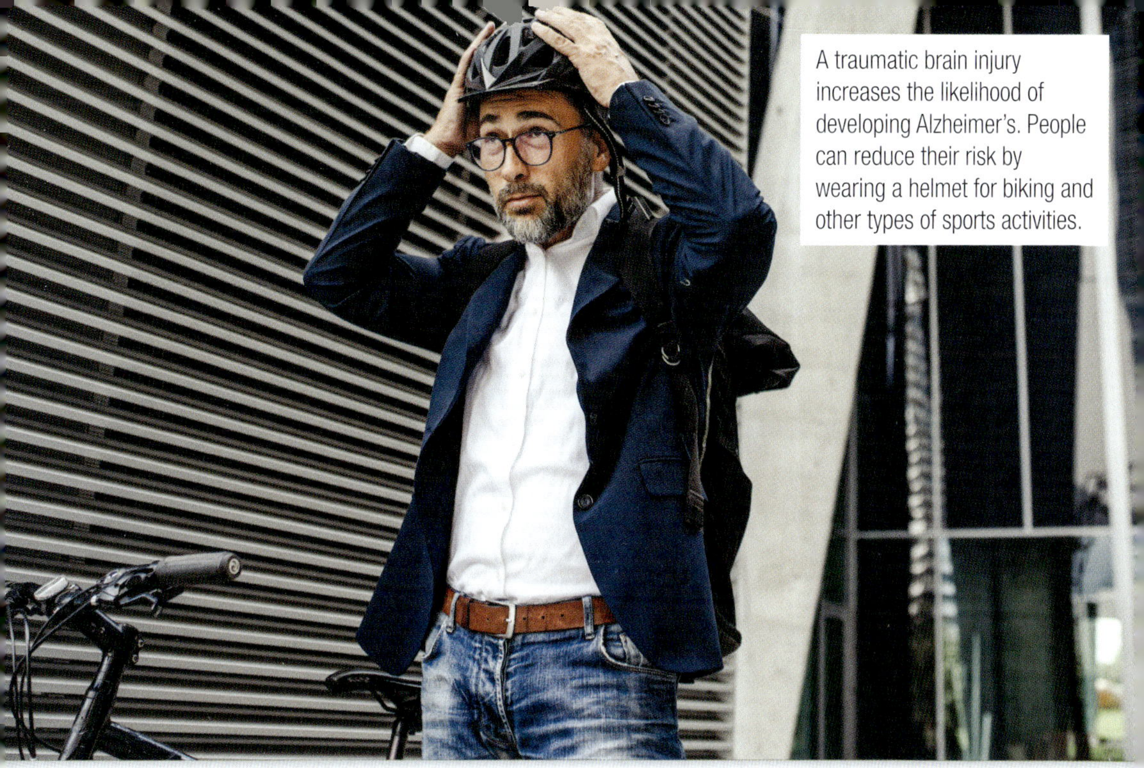

A traumatic brain injury increases the likelihood of developing Alzheimer's. People can reduce their risk by wearing a helmet for biking and other types of sports activities.

who have hearing loss later in life also have a higher risk of Alzheimer's. Another type of injury associated with Alzheimer's is traumatic brain injury. Again, researchers do not fully understand the connection between the two. They theorize that a brain injury somehow affects the brain's ability to fight off the development of plaques and tangles.

Smoking and Drinking

Finally, researchers also believe that smoking and drinking increase the risk of developing Alzheimer's disease. The American Heart Association reports that smokers are 40 percent more likely to get Alzheimer's disease, with the risk increasing with the amount they smoke. Jennifer Deal, an assistant professor of epidemiology at the Johns Hopkins Bloomberg School of Public Health in Baltimore, led a study on the relationship between smoking and dementia. She notes that for those who have been smokers, quitting smoking can significantly decrease the risk. "The message coming out of our research is that earlier is better," Deal says, "Quitting in midlife is better than later in life. But quitting at any time is beneficial."[18]

“It is clear that excessive drinking increases a person’s risk of dementia compared with not drinking at all.”[19]

—Alzheimer’s Society

According to the Alzheimer’s Society, heavy alcohol consumption also makes developing Alzheimer’s more likely. According to the society, “It is clear that excessive drinking increases a person’s risk of dementia compared with not drinking at all.”[19] The Alzheimer’s Society explains that research studies have shown that people who drink heavily are more likely to develop dementia than those who are not heavy drinkers. Experts do not understand exactly how alcohol consumption increases the risk of Alzheimer’s, but they think that drinking causes changes in the brain that can lead to the disease.

Reducing the Risk of Alzheimer’s

There is no sure way to completely eliminate the risk of developing Alzheimer’s, since researchers still do not completely understand why this disease develops in the first place. However, because many risk factors have been identified, it is possible for people to reduce the likelihood of developing Alzheimer’s by making some lifestyle changes. The CDC suggests five lifestyle habits that can lower the risk of Alzheimer’s and other dementias: staying physically active, preventing or managing diabetes, maintaining a healthy blood pressure, limiting smoking or drinking, and preventing or correcting hearing loss. With habits such as these, the CDC says, “Nearly 45% of all dementia cases may be prevented or delayed.”[20] Other expert suggestions for reducing the risk of Alzheimer’s include getting enough sleep, staying socially active, eating a healthy diet, and wearing a helmet for sports activities like biking, skating, and skiing to protect from head trauma.

There is also evidence that people can help protect themselves against Alzheimer’s by building something called cognitive reserve, which is the ability to retain cognitive function even when the brain is damaged. The brain naturally grows and changes throughout a person’s lifetime, in response to many different factors such as environment, health, social life, and mental stimulation, making new connections when presented with challenges and losing connections when cells die because of illness. Researchers think that when a person stimulates their brain by learning new things and being socially engaged, they build cognitive reserve, meaning that their brain becomes more resistant to anything that might threaten its function. They believe that when a person with cognitive reserve experiences the brain changes caused by Alzheimer's, that reserve allows them to keep functioning normally. In support of this theory, researchers have found that there are some people who have the brain changes associated with Alzheimer's but do not display symptoms of the disease. These scientists theorize that cognitive reserve has allowed such individuals to keep functioning normally despite the physical changes in the brain.

The Challenge of Understanding the Brain

Every year, an enormous amount of time and money is devoted to better understanding Alzheimer's disease, but this has proved to be a challenging field of research. Part of the challenge comes from the fact that researchers do not fully understand the human brain itself. The complexity of the brain, with its billions of neurons and trillions of synapses, makes Alzheimer's research challenging. As Alzheimer's researcher Donald Weaver explains, "The human brain is extremely complex, and Alzheimer's disease is one of the most complex diseases of the brain." However, scientists like Weaver are optimistic that human beings' incredible brain power will eventually be used to solve this puzzle. Says Weaver, "We'll get there."[21]

> "The human brain is extremely complex, and Alzheimer's disease is one of the most complex diseases of the brain."[21]
>
> —Donald Weaver, Alzheimer's researcher

How Alzheimer's Is Diagnosed and Treated

When Nancy started experiencing memory problems that seemed like they might be early symptoms of Alzheimer's disease, she did not wait for things to get worse. Instead, she looked for expert diagnosis and treatment. A brain specialist evaluated her symptoms and diagnosed her with Alzheimer's. She started treatment with a drug called lecanemab, which has been shown to reduce cognitive decline in some people who are in the early stages of the disease. Nancy recognizes that her disease is irreversible and incurable, but she hopes that by starting treatment early, she can stop it from getting worse. She says:

> I'm willing to try anything. I know I won't get my brain back, but I've got to stop this where it is. . . . I want to still be able to drive. And remember names and birthdays. I love working in the garden and watching birds. We have a group of five women. We call ourselves "The Divas." We go out to dinner and celebrate birthdays. . . . And I go to Pilates on Wednesdays. . . . I don't want to lose those kinds of things.[22]

While there is currently no cure for Alzheimer's disease, research has led to the development of a number of drug treatments that can slow the progression of this disease for some people and help with their symptoms. Because a person's existing symptoms cannot be reversed, doctors stress that early diagnosis and treatment are important; the sooner treatment starts, the more likely it is that a person can live for longer without more serious symptoms.

Diagnosing Alzheimer's

If a person is worried that they might have Alzheimer's, the first step is usually to visit a doctor. There is no single definitive test that can determine whether someone has Alzheimer's. Instead, doctors use a variety of information to decide whether Alzheimer's is the likely cause. According to Johns Hopkins Medicine, in most cases this detective work leads to an accurate diagnosis. "Specialists can rule out other similar conditions and diagnose Alzheimer's disease with about 95 percent accuracy,"[23] says the institution. However, the only way to confirm the presence of the disease for sure is by examining brain tissue after a patient dies.

> "Specialists can rule out other similar conditions and diagnose Alzheimer's disease with about 95 percent accuracy."[23]
>
> —Johns Hopkins Medicine

When diagnosing Alzheimer's, doctors usually start by asking about a person's symptoms and their general health. They might conduct tests to evaluate memory, thinking, and problem-solving, since problems with any of these functions are possible indications of Alzheimer's. A doctor will also likely order blood work and other medical tests to rule out other conditions such as a thyroid problem or some kind of infection. In some cases they may even do brain imaging—like a magnetic resonance imaging, computed tomography, or positron-emission tomography (PET) scan—which can also help them rule out other causes such as a tumor or bleeding in the brain.

Brain imaging can also be used specifically to look for evidence that is highly suggestive of Alzheimer's. People with this disease have a buildup of the protein beta-amyloid in their brain, which might be visible with a PET scan. In some cases doctors also look for the presence of beta-amyloid by testing a person's spinal fluid.

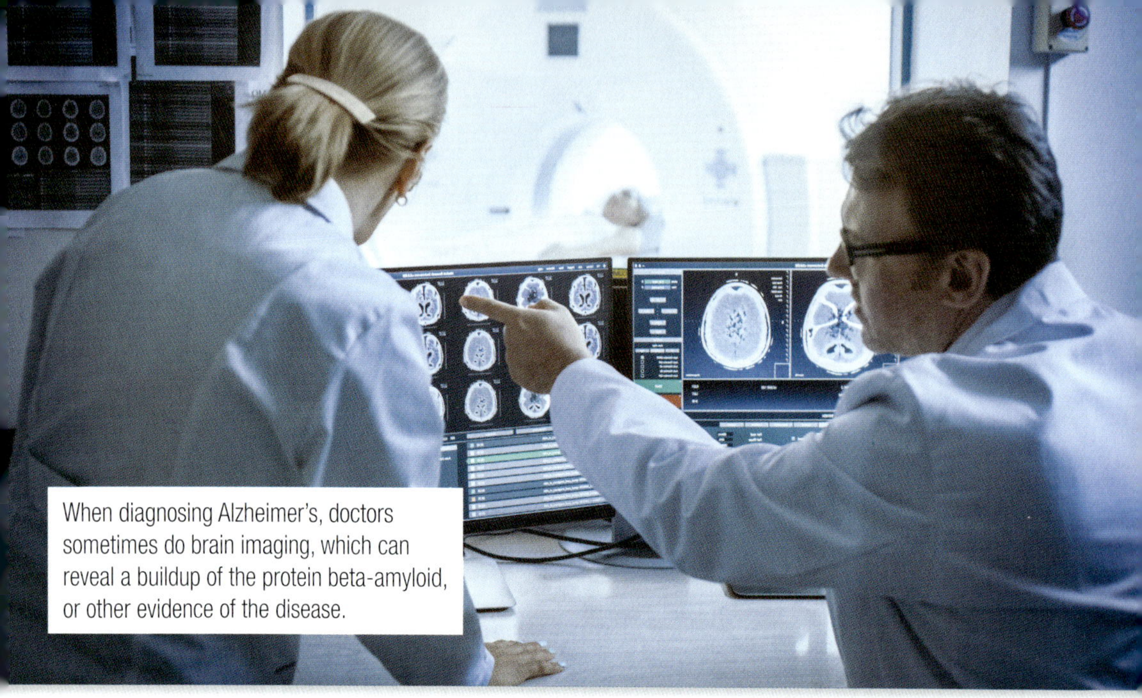

When diagnosing Alzheimer's, doctors sometimes do brain imaging, which can reveal a buildup of the protein beta-amyloid, or other evidence of the disease.

An Emphasis on Early Diagnosis

In recent years there has been a lot of focus on developing better diagnostic tools for Alzheimer's because early diagnosis often allows doctors to treat the disease more effectively and possibly slow it down. Mayo Clinic authors Jonathan Graff-Radford and Angela M. Lunde explain that there are numerous benefits to being diagnosed while symptoms are still mild. "You may be a candidate for medication that can lessen symptoms and slow progression of the disease," they say. "An early diagnosis also allows families the opportunity to understand the disease, know what to expect, and learn how to adapt, cope and gain access to resources. All of this can make it easier to manage Alzheimer's symptoms."[24]

"An early diagnosis . . . allows families the opportunity to understand the disease, know what to expect, and learn how to adapt, cope and gain access to resources. All of this can make it easier to manage Alzheimer's symptoms."[24]

—Jonathan Graff-Radford and Angela M. Lunde, authors of *Mayo Clinic on Alzheimer's Disease and Other Dementias*

In 2025 the US Food and Drug Administration (FDA) approved the first blood test for Alzheimer's, and scientists hope that this will be an important step in helping more people get an early diagnosis. The test looks for the presence of beta-amyloid and tau, two proteins that build up in the brain when a person has Alzheimer's disease. Combined with other patient information, this blood test can help doctors diagnose Alzheimer's. Blood tests are a relatively new tool and not yet widely used, but researchers hope that they will become more common and more accurate in the future because such tests are cheaper and less invasive than other testing options such taking spinal fluid or doing a brain scan.

Drug Treatment for Alzheimer's

Most people who are diagnosed with Alzheimer's receive some type of drug treatment. There are two main types of drugs for this disease: those that temporarily slow its progression and those that help alleviate some of its symptoms. For drugs that slow progression, two have been approved by the FDA for use in the United States: donanemab (brand name Kisunla) and lecanemab (brand name Leqembi). These drugs work by removing beta-amyloid from the brain. They do not help everyone, but there is evidence that for some people they are very effective, particularly if they are started in the early stages of the disease. Larry, who lives in the United Kingdom—where lecanemab has also been approved—started taking the drug after his early diagnosis of Alzheimer's. He says that it has helped slow memory loss significantly, stating, "On lecanemab [my memory] hasn't slipped a lot further. I've taken memory tests every six months and those really

Cognitive Testing

When a person visits a doctor because they are worried about whether they have Alzheimer's disease, that doctor is likely to perform a screening test to evaluate their cognition, such as their memory, thinking, and problem-solving abilities. Some tests can be completed quickly, while others are more time-consuming, but they are all designed to help doctors understand whether a person is experiencing any cognitive problems. Commonly used tests such as the Mini-Mental State Examination and the Montreal Cognitive Assessment ask patients to do things like remember a list of words, perform simple calculations, and follow instructions for basic tasks. These tests have a relatively high level of accuracy in screening for dementia, but are less helpful in determining whether the cause of that dementia is Alzheimer's or something else.

haven't changed in the time I've been on the trial. . . . I am still able to live a full life—going on bike rides, playing mahjong, and socialising with friends and family."[25]

There are also drugs that help alleviate some of the symptoms that people with Alzheimer's experience. The FDA has approved a number of drugs that can help stabilize the cognitive problems that occur with the disease. These drugs do not stop the Alzheimer's from progressing, but they can temporarily improve things like memory, attention, and cognition. They do this by influencing the chemicals in the brain that help its cells communicate with one another. Drugs in this category include donepezil, galantamine, and memantine. In addition to drugs that treat their cognitive symptoms, some Alzheimer's patients take medications that help them with some of the other—noncognitive—symptoms that can come with this disease. For instance, they might take an anti-insomnia medicine if they are experiencing trouble sleeping or an antipsychotic drug to reduce agitation or hallucinations.

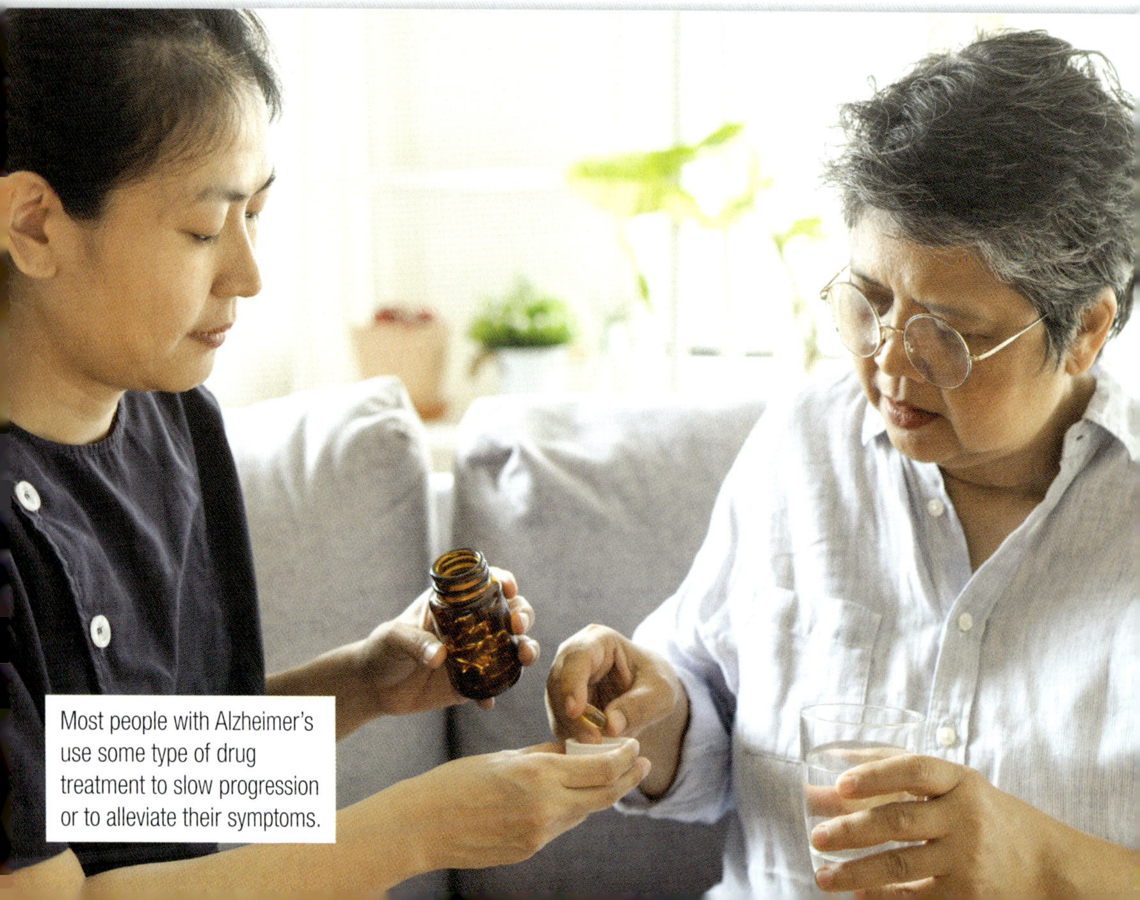

Most people with Alzheimer's use some type of drug treatment to slow progression or to alleviate their symptoms.

Dietary Supplements and Herbal Treatments

Many dietary supplements and herbal treatments are promoted as treatments for Alzheimer's disease, including ginkgo biloba and omega-3 fatty acids. However, most experts express caution when it comes to such alternative treatments. The Alzheimer's Association insists that there is no evidence that these treatments work. "Not a single food, beverage, ingredient, vitamin or supplement has been proven to prevent, treat or cure Alzheimer's disease or to benefit cognitive function or brain health." In addition, Alzheimer's Association experts warn that many supplements are unregulated and can actually have harmful side effects.

Alzheimer's Association, "Alternative Treatments," 2025. www.alz.org.

While drugs are helpful for many people, Alzheimer's is still challenging to treat. Doctors explain that treatment is an ongoing process of working with patients to evaluate the progression of the disease, understand how well treatment is working, and revise the treatment plan if necessary. Graff-Radford and Lunde stress, "The one constant with the disease often is change. Symptoms may change, fluctuate, go away or intensify. In response, treatment and care must be adapted or refined."[26]

Other Types of Treatment

Drugs are not the only treatment option for Alzheimer's disease. Most patients also try other strategies to help alleviate the symptoms of the disease and improve their quality of life. In fact, the Alzheimer's Association insists, "non-drug approaches should always be tried first."[27] Many nondrug approaches involve working to understand the root cause of the symptom a person is experience and trying to address that cause. For instance, a person with Alzheimer's might be agitated or have trouble sleeping, and investigation might reveal that this is because there is a new caregiving arrangement. Addressing that change, such as trying to help the person feel more comfortable with the new caregiver or caregiving routine, might reduce agitation or difficulty sleeping.

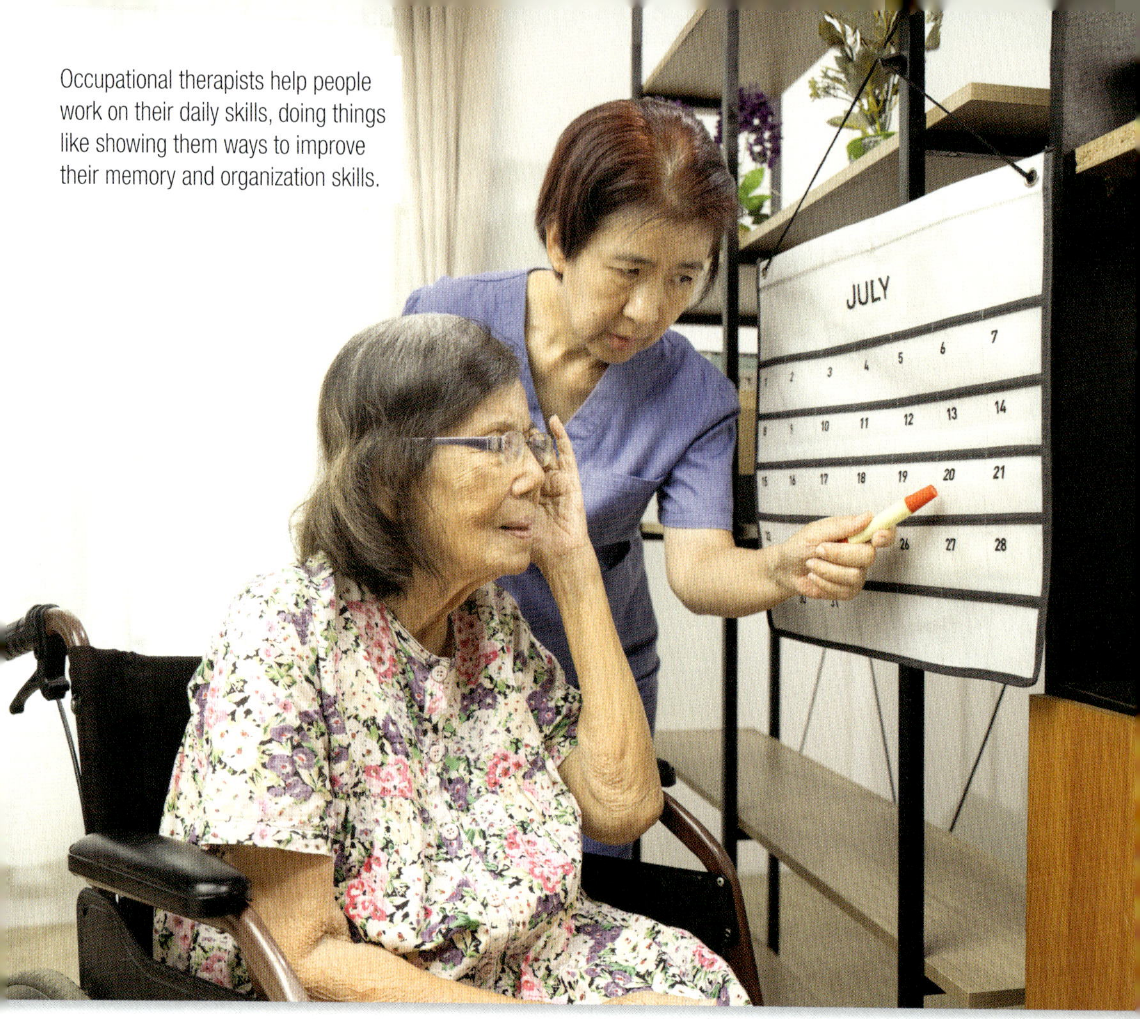

Occupational therapists help people work on their daily skills, doing things like showing them ways to improve their memory and organization skills.

Many people with Alzheimer's also receive occupational therapy, which is designed to improve their quality of life. Occupational therapists help people work on daily skills like dressing, personal hygiene, and eating. They recommend changes to the home, like adding grab bars or a shower chair to prevent falls or improving organization to reduce confusion. They might also suggest strategies like music therapy to help manage anxiety or behavioral problems. The goal of occupational therapy is to help a person with Alzheimer's live independently and safely as long as they can. Occupational therapists may also work with family members or caregivers to help them understand how best to support and care for the person with Alzheimer's.

Willy lives in Edinburgh, Scotland, and receives regular occupational therapy for his Alzheimer's disease. He explains that his therapist works with him to understand his unique challenges, like remembering where to find his art supplies, and come up with solutions for those challenges. For instance, he says, "I now keep a record each day and this isn't something historically I have done. But I have started to realise this really is important, and if I don't note down where I've been and what I've been up to, I do start to lose track. I also organise my art materials with labels and put things away in the right slots. I know it sounds silly as a grown man, but it really has helped."[28]

Caring for People with Alzheimer's

Even with treatment, people with Alzheimer's eventually start needing help with daily tasks. For most people, help comes from caregivers who assist with things like bathing, grooming, house-cleaning, shopping, and meal preparation. Depending on how much help is needed, a caregiver might visit for a certain number of hours every day or week, or the person with Alzheimer's might live with a caregiver or have the caregiver live with them. According to the CDC, about 80 percent of adults with Alzheimer's disease and related dementias receive care in their home. A lot of this care comes from friends and family members. However, some people get help from paid caregivers.

As the disease progresses, some people require constant care and may need to move to a dedicated care facility that specializes in providing around-the-clock care for people with Alzheimer's or other types of dementia. A Harvard Health article explains that this type of facility can be beneficial because it is run by experts who know how to deal with this disease. The author says, "Memory care offers a safe and secure environment, with staff members trained to calm and reassure people with dementia-related changes in mood, behavior, and personality, such as increased anxiety or irritability. They offer a structured environment and activities to help residents feel connected and valued as their disease progresses."[29] However, most care facilities are expensive, and this option is unaffordable for many people. According to the Alzheimer's Association, an assisted living facility costs about $70,000 per year. This type of facility is for people who need some help with everyday tasks but do not need full-time care. A semiprivate room in a nursing home that provides a much higher level of supervision and medical care costs on average about $111,000 a year.

Hope for the Future

All over the world, an enormous amount of research is being focused on Alzheimer's. Scientists are working to get a better understanding of what causes the disease, how to treat it more effectively, and ultimately, how to prevent or cure it. While a cure remains elusive, there have been many advances in understanding and treatment in recent years. Specifically, researchers have developed more effective drugs and improved diagnosis and testing methods. For instance, some researchers are using artificial intelligence (AI) to improve treatment by diagnosing Alzheimer's sooner. World Economic Forum writer Madeleine North explains that in a University of California study, researchers were able to use AI to predict the development of Alzheimer's up to seven years before the appearance of symptoms and were accurate 72 percent of the time. In a study at Cambridge University in the United Kingdom, she says, researchers predicted the speed of cognitive impairment developing and had an 81 percent accuracy rate. North quotes UK researcher Zoe Kourtzi, who insists, "This has the potential to significantly improve patient wellbeing, showing us which people need closest care, while removing the anxiety for those patients we predict will remain stable."[30]

> "There's a lot of work to do and a long way to go. But we can see a very different future for people living with dementia, and one day, a cure."[31]
>
> —Susan Kohlhaas, executive director of research at Alzheimer's Research UK

Susan Kohlhaas, executive director of research at Alzheimer's Research UK, insists that with researchers making many significant breakthroughs in recent years, there is real hope that there will one day be a cure for this disease. She argues that the recently developed drugs that slow cognitive decline suggest there is a way to cure Alzheimer's. She says:

> Lecanemab and donanemab are a huge leap forward. They are the first treatments that can slow memory and thinking decline linked to Alzheimer's, rather than just alleviating symptoms. . . . They open the door to future treatments that will be safer and more effective, bringing us closer to a day when we can slow, stop, and even reverse all forms of dementia, keeping us connected with our loved ones for longer. . . . There's a lot of work to do and a long way to go. But we can see a very different future for people living with dementia, and one day, a cure.[31]

Chapter Four

How Alzheimer's Disease Affects People and Their Families

Alzheimer's disease is life-altering both for the person who has it and for their family and friends. Janice talks about what happened after her mom, Gabriella, started showing the symptoms of this disease. She says, "It changed our lives in ways that we could have never imagined. This lovely lady who took pride in her family, her home, her garden, and who enjoyed shopping, doing her hair, nails, and makeup, watching TV, reading, playing Bingo, cooking, and cleaning—yes, she even enjoyed cleaning—slowly ceased to exist." Janice describes some of the ways that her mom changed: "She began to lose interest in many of the things she loved to do—the things we loved to do together. She no longer recognized her home, she often didn't recognize me, her only daughter, her only child. There were times when my mom was agitated and combative. She would hear and see things that we couldn't see. She would say the most hurtful and heartbreaking things to me."[32] People with Alzheimer's, and those close to them, say that changes like this are both emotionally wrenching and extremely challenging to deal with.

What It Feels like to Have Alzheimer's

For those diagnosed with Alzheimer's, one of the saddest things about their illness is what it takes away. Patients gradually lose their memories, the capacity to take part in the activities they have always enjoyed, and eventually their ability to live in their own home or even care for themselves on a basic level. Rick

Phelps, who has early-onset Alzheimer's disease, explains that this loss is a gradual but sure process. He says, "This condition only takes a little from you at first—a few of your short-term memories here and there. Then, slowly but surely, it takes all of them. In time, it begins to steal your long-term memories as well. Eventually, they will all be gone." The realization that all of this is disappearing is terrifying, he explains. Equally terrifying is the fact that he knows he is powerless to stop it. He says, "All along, you realize that this is happening, but there isn't a single thing you can do about it. I often think about what will happen when I can no longer remember who I am or who those around me are. What will it be like? Will I be scared? More scared than I am now at times? Is that even possible?"[33]

> "I often think about what will happen when I can no longer remember who I am or who those around me are. What will it be like? Will I be scared? More scared than I am now at times? Is that even possible?"[33]
>
> —Rick Phelps, who has early-onset Alzheimer's disease

As they lose their memories and ability to accomplish tasks, people with Alzheimer's are forced to change the way they live. Peter has Alzheimer's and discusses some of the things he does differently now. He says, "With money, I know what a coin looks like but can't add them up anymore. I have no idea how to do it. I get round it by using contactless cards."[34] In addition, he says that he no longer reads very much because he keeps forgetting what he just read. He enjoys watching television but has switched to wildlife documentaries because with other types of shows, he keeps losing the plot.

As more and more abilities are lost, people with Alzheimer's' start needing help with so many everyday tasks—like shopping and feeding and bathing themselves—that they also lose their independence. They can no longer look after themselves and are forced to rely on regular help from caregivers.

Negative Emotions

The loss of abilities and independence and the change in lifestyle that come with Alzheimer's often cause negative emotions, including frustration, anger, anxiety, and depression. There is a long list of reasons that an Alzheimer's patient might experience these emotions. It can be distressing to forget things or not understand what is happening and frustrating to be unable to do certain things or communicate effectively. Individuals may also feel worried about what is happening to them, or anxious and unhappy because of loneliness or boredom. Some people with Alzheimer's also feel like they are being forced to do things they do not want to do, such as visit the doctor or make changes to their lifestyle, which can make them feel angry. Experts think that some of these negative emotions are not just a result of frustration or anxiety but come from the changes that Alzheimer's causes in the brain.

In some cases these negative emotions may become extreme, and a person with Alzheimer's might yell and threaten other people or become physically aggressive; for instance, biting, scratching, or throwing things. Commenting on an Alzheimer's Society Facebook post, Cheryl Liddell talks about a violent incident that

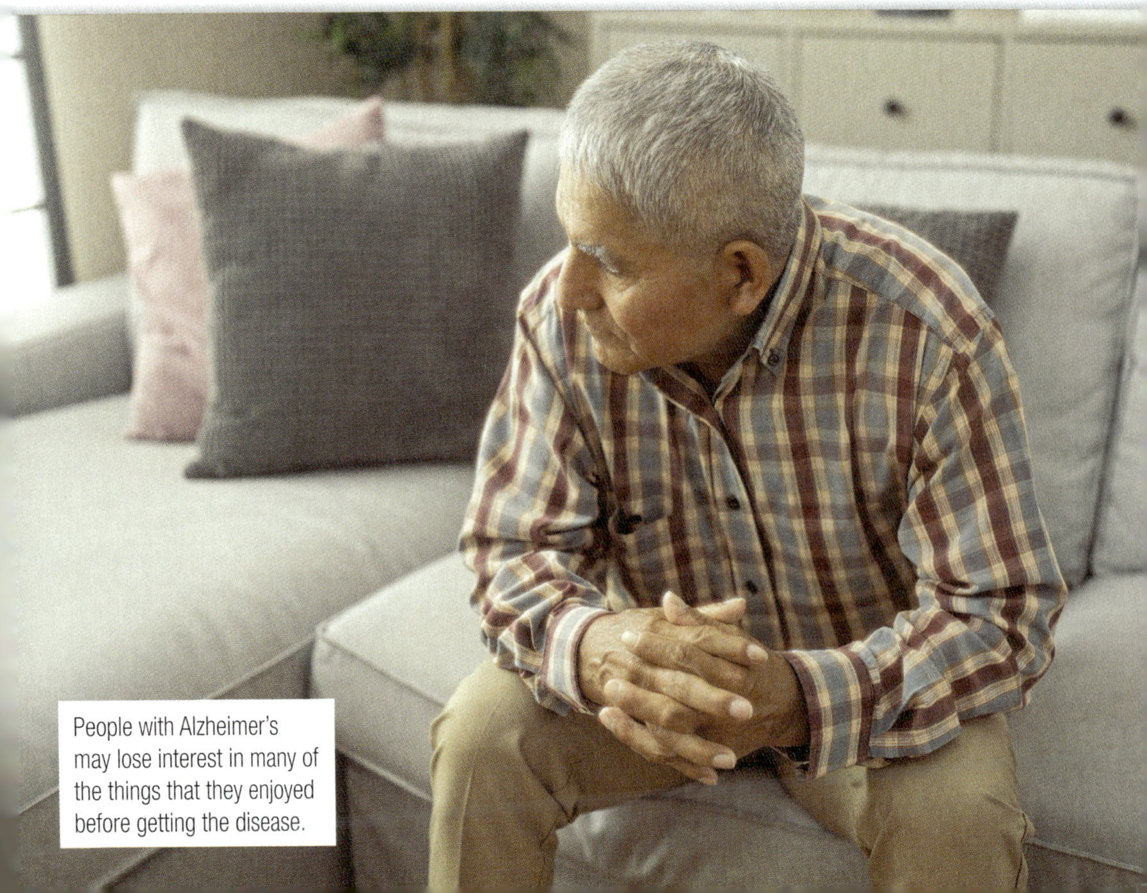

People with Alzheimer's may lose interest in many of the things that they enjoyed before getting the disease.

happened on Christmas Day. She explains that after having her mother at her house, she took her back to her mother's own home, which was nearby. However, her mother instantly wanted to leave again and became angry when Lidell tried to calm her down. Liddell recalls, "She bit my hand then put her hands round my throat and I couldn't breathe. It was the most horrific and frightening experience of my life as she was always so loving. I walked away in bits."[35]

Friends and Family Members

As Liddell's story reveals, not only is Alzheimer's frightening for those people who have it, but dealing with this disease is also a challenging experience for friends and family members. Katie Stevens was fifteen when her grandmother was diagnosed with Alzheimer's disease. She explains that it is difficult to understand just how challenging Alzheimer's is without experiencing it in real life. She says, "I knew about [Alzheimer's] from friends . . . but nothing can ever prepare you for what comes after the diagnosis."[36] She explains that she was stunned at how much suffering her grandmother went through as she lost her memory and her ability to look after herself. In addition, she says, the family suffered as they watched her grandmother deteriorate.

> "I will always love my grandad and I will treasure all the memories we've had together, but sadly he is no longer the man he used to be, and the saddest part is that man is never coming back."[37]
>
> —Lizzie Thomson, whose grandfather has Alzheimer's

Many people talk about how sad it is to see Alzheimer's change their loved one, taking away a vibrant personality and leaving that person confused and afraid. Lizzie Thomson explains that Alzheimer's completely changed her grandfather. She says, "My grandad was like a father figure to me growing up. Now at 93, after a few years of suffering with Alzheimer's disease, very little of his charismatic personality is left. I will always love my grandad and I will treasure all the memories we've had together, but sadly he is no longer the man he used to be, and the saddest part is that man is never coming back."[37] Judy

Understanding What It Feels Like

Rick Phelps has early-onset Alzheimer's disease. He insists, "I think it is important for people to understand what dementia patients truly go through instead of relying on expert speculations." To help with this, he offers an imaginary scenario that illustrates just how confusing this disease can feel. To start with, he says, imagine giving a person a drug that puts them to sleep and takes away their ability to make short-term memories. Next, he says:

> Have them awaken in a building they have never been in before that is full of furniture and items they do not recognize. . . . One by one, have complete strangers enter the room and talk to the person as if they have known each other their entire lives. Have these strangers talk to the person as if each one of them is their daughter, their spouse or their pastor. . . . The entire time, this person will be wondering what in the world is going on.

Rick Phelps, "What It Really Feels like to Have Alzheimer's Disease," AgingCare, 2025. www.agingcare.com.

Born says the same thing about her husband Doug, "It's hard to watch somebody just disappear," she says, "And that's what he's doing—he's disappearing."[38]

Being a Caregiver

Because Alzheimer's is such a common disease, the number of people who find themselves becoming caregivers to afflicted family members is immense. According to the Alzheimer's Association, in the United States more than 11 million people serve as unpaid caregivers for someone with Alzheimer's or another type of dementia. About two-thirds of caregivers are women. Young people often find themselves in caregiving roles too. The American Association of Caregiving Youth reports that more than 5 million people age eighteen or younger provide a substantial amount of care for a family member who has a significant medical condition like Alzheimer's.

Being a caregiver is not easy. It is both emotionally and physically taxing. Alzheimer's patients often need constant care and attention, leaving caregivers little time to focus on their own health and well-being. Karen Mack is a caregiver for both of her parents, who still live in their own home in Los Angeles but who need constant care. Karen and her sister share the caregiving duties, spending alternate nights sleeping at their parents' house and looking after them. "Having to sleep over there is very difficult," she says. "My mom doesn't sleep. . . . Then I have to come and do a full day of work." She says that caregiving is overwhelming: "I'm trying to manage two households. I'm buying groceries, medications, [making] doctor appointments, paying their bills, doing their taxes. I do everything. It's an energy drain. . . . Also, I'm not here for my family. My house is a disaster because I don't have the energy to clean it."[39]

Researchers find that Alzheimer's caregivers report a high rate of stress and are also much more likely to suffer from depression than people who are not caregivers. In many cases these issues are ignored, because the needs of the caregiver are overshadowed by the needs of the person they are caring for.

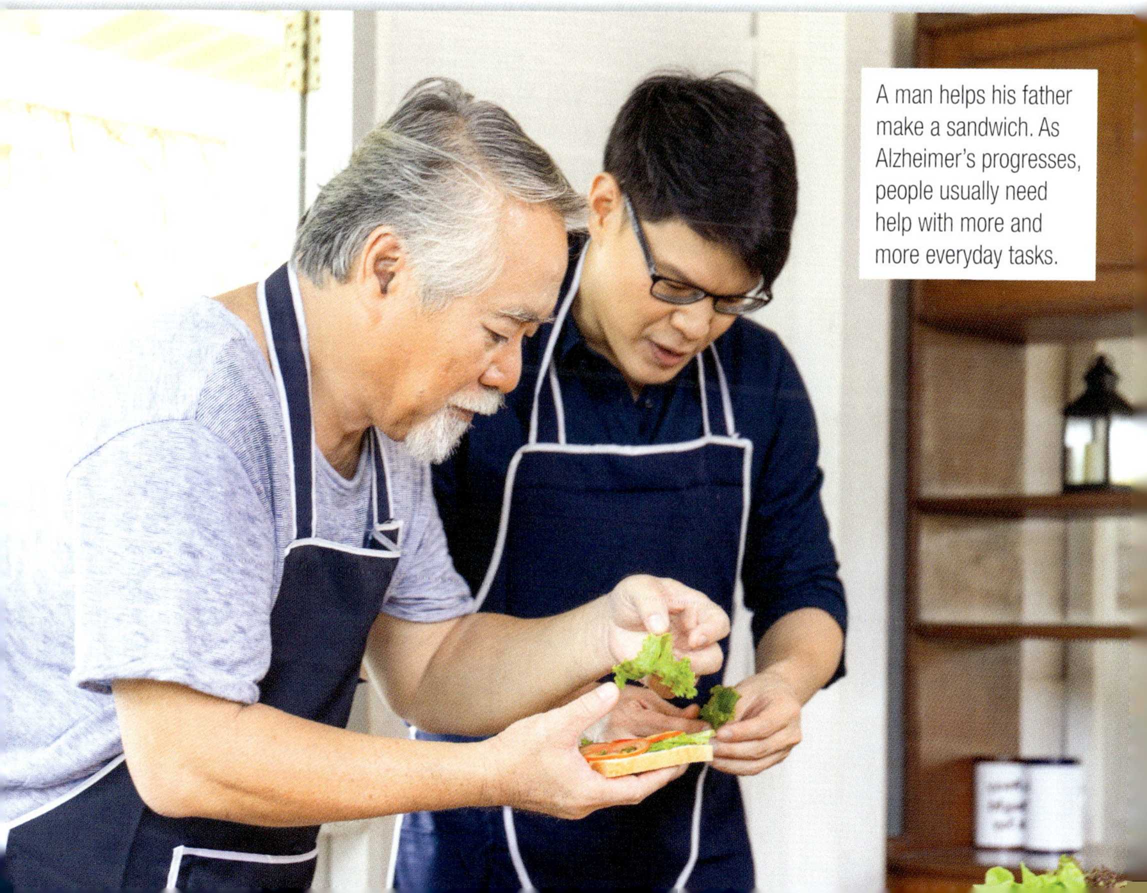

A man helps his father make a sandwich. As Alzheimer's progresses, people usually need help with more and more everyday tasks.

In addition to often working day and night, caregivers often receive very little gratitude for what they do and may even be treated poorly by the person they are trying to care for. Alzheimer's patients may get angry with their caregiver, say mean things to them, or not recognize them. Cameron Huddleston talks about caring for her mom, who never talks to her except when she is unhappy about something. She says that once, after taking her to a doctor's appointment, her mom refused to leave with her at the end of the appointment. Another time, she says that her mom needed surgery, and "I had to hold her arms in the recovery room to prevent her from yanking her IV out. She called me names. She tried to hit and bite me. I was only trying to help her, but my mom thought I was trying to hurt her."[40]

Alzheimer's and Stigma

People with Alzheimer's, caregivers, and friends and family members are also affected by the stigma associated with this disease. There are many negative beliefs and stereotypes associated with Alzheimer's disease, in addition to a general lack of understanding about what it involves, and this means that people who have Alzheimer's are often treated in ways that are discriminatory, demeaning, or unkind. One example is making assumptions about what a person with Alzheimer's can or cannot do and acting based on those assumptions. For example, someone might talk about

Importance of Self-Care for Caregivers

Being a caregiver for someone with Alzheimer's can be challenging. Experts stress that it is vitally important for every caregiver to take time to look after themselves too. To many caregivers, self-care is a lesser priority. The National Institute on Aging explains, "You may feel that you should be able to do everything yourself, that it's not okay for you to leave the person you're caring for with someone else, or that none of your friends and family would help if you asked." However, the agency insists that neglecting this important area can lead to illness or depression. The agency suggests asking friends and family members for help or getting expert help from a home care agency or adult day care service.

National Institute on Aging, "Alzheimer's Caregiving: Caring for Yourself," July 11, 2024. www.nia.nih.gov.

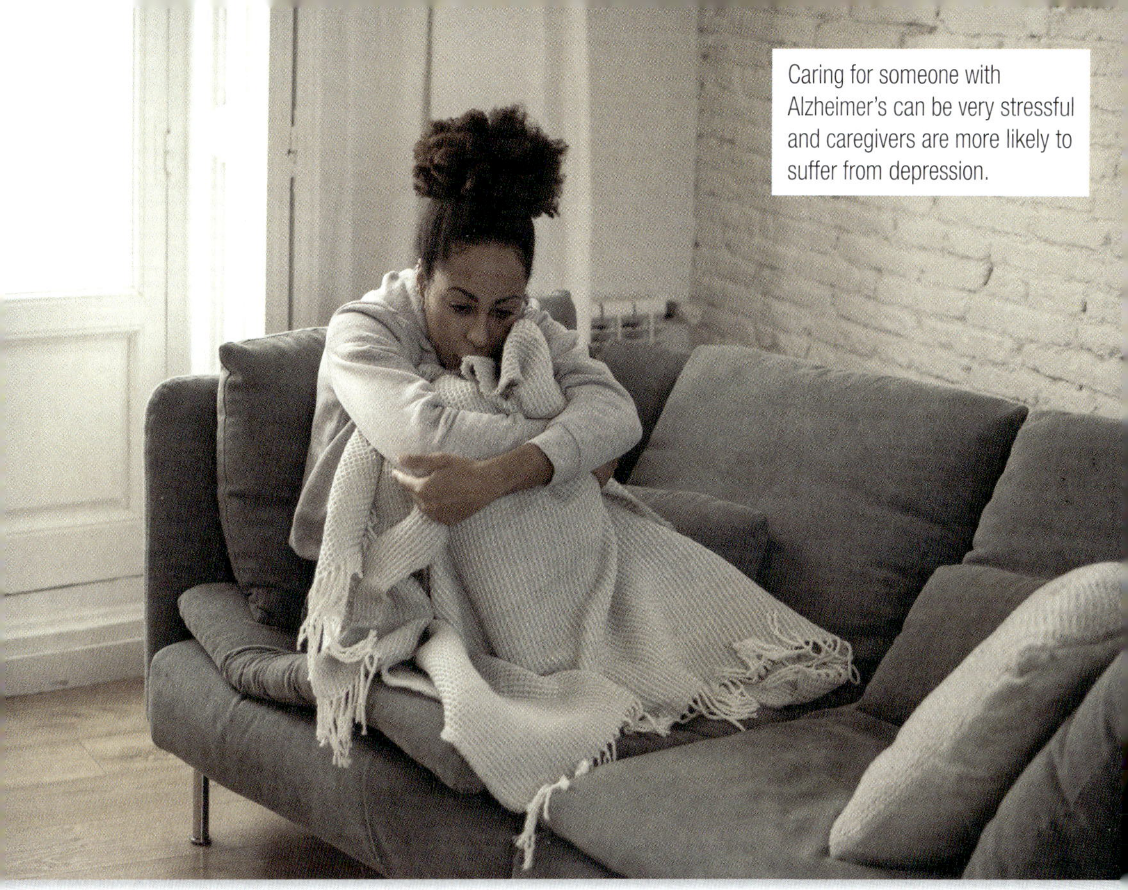

Caring for someone with Alzheimer's can be very stressful and caregivers are more likely to suffer from depression.

the individual as if they are incompetent or not present, when they are actually right there and able to speak for themselves. Another example is making jokes or using negative language. The Alzheimer's Society of Canada explains some common types of negative language associated with Alzheimer's disease. "Negative language is often used to describe dementia, tending to focus on the losses brought on by the disease—for example, 'people *suffering* with dementia.'" In addition, how a person with Alzheimer's is referred to may be considered hurtful. "Wording can also reduce the experiences of people living with dementia to a series of labels, symptoms or medical terms. No one wants to be considered a 'patient' or a 'case' of Alzheimer's disease."[41]

In an article in the *AMA Journal of Ethics*, three experts on aging share stories from some people who have Alzheimer's and have experienced stigma. One person says, "People didn't know how to talk to me even though I was the same person I was five minutes before I told them I had it. They just saw this big A on my forehead. They didn't look at me as the same person—I was stupid, or couldn't carry a conversation, or have a single thought of my own, which was very distressing to me."[42]

Stigma has a lot of negative consequences. For example, stigma often prevents people from seeking a diagnosis to begin with. Avoiding diagnosis is harmful because it delays treatment, meaning that the disease progresses more quickly and a person deteriorates faster. Not getting a diagnosis also makes it more difficult to get support or to plan for the future. Another impact of Alzheimer's stigma is that it often causes other people to avoid those who have Alzheimer's because they feel uncomfortable or unsure of how to act around them. Finally, it can make people feel ashamed for having a disease that is not their fault, and this can cause them to withdraw and avoid social interaction.

Still a Person

Alzheimer's is challenging both for those who have it and for their friends and family. However, people who have experienced this devastating disease stress that despite the challenges, it is important to remember that having Alzheimer's does not take away a person's need to be treated with dignity and respect. Lindsey Ko is a teenager whose great uncle was diagnosed with Alzheimer's. She says, "I wish others would know that although Alzheimer's disease does impact the actions of the affected individual, it doesn't make them any less of who they are. A person with Alzheimer's disease is still a person, and they deserve the same interactions, respect, and empathy as someone without the disease."[43]

"A person with Alzheimer's disease is still a person, and they deserve the same interactions, respect, and empathy as someone without the disease."[43]

—Lindsey Ko, a teenager whose great uncle was diagnosed with Alzheimer's

Chapter Five

Ways to Connect with People Who Have Alzheimer's

The internet is full of stories from people whose friends or family members have Alzheimer's disease. They share their experiences and often ask for advice. One thing that many people ask about is how to connect with someone who has changed because of Alzheimer's. For instance, on one discussion forum, a user writes that she is struggling to deal with the way that her grandmother has become different as her disease has progressed. She explains:

> My grandma had been diagnosed with Alzheimer's a few months back. Recently it has gotten worse. Yesterday I helped my mom and her aunt move my grandma's stuff into her new care home. It was my first time seeing my grandma since the Alzheimer's got worse. It was really hard for me to see her like that and I spent most of the day crying and holding her hand. What can I do to comfort her and tell her I love and care about her?[44]

While Alzheimer's affects everyone differently, one certainty is that it causes change. A person with this disease might act differently, not enjoy doing the same things they once did, have trouble communicating, or even not recognize someone they have known for years. With all these changes, it can be more challenging for friends and family members to connect with someone with Alzheimer's. However, it is important to know that connection is still possible.

Communication Difficulties

Experts explain that one reason connection can be challenging is that Alzheimer's makes it more difficult for a person to communicate. They might have trouble remembering words and organizing them into logical sentences, remembering what was said, or even knowing who they are talking to. All these things make it much more challenging to have a two-way conversation. However, this difficulty does not diminish the need for communication. Every human being—including Alzheimer's patients—needs human communication and connection. Connection with other peo-

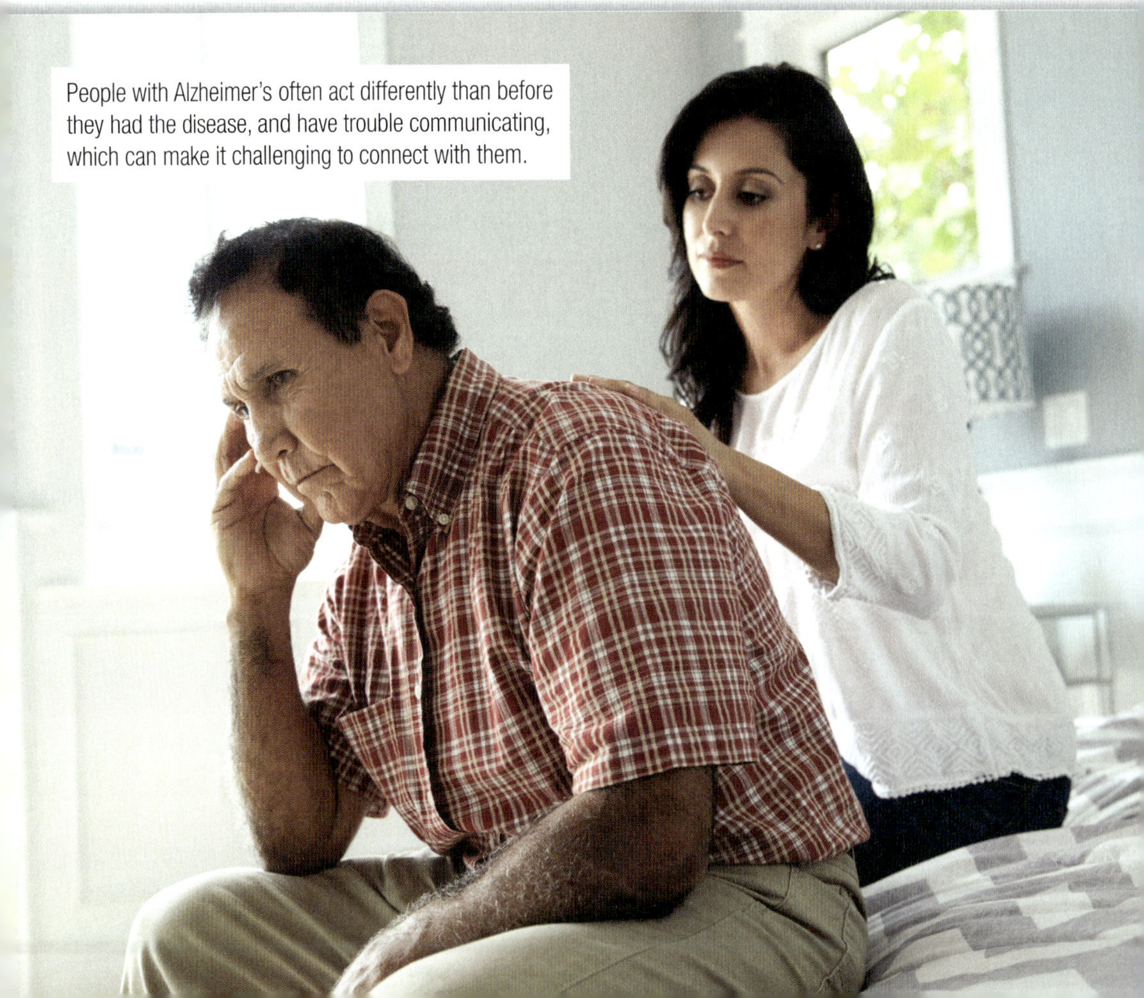

People with Alzheimer's often act differently than before they had the disease, and have trouble communicating, which can make it challenging to connect with them.

ple improves emotional well-being and gives a sense of belonging and purpose. For people with Alzheimer's, a sense of connection can help them feel happier and less lonely or anxious. There is also evidence that connection can help preserve cognitive function and slow the progression of the disease.

Experts offer a few different strategies for successful communication with a person who has Alzheimer's. First, they stress that it is important not to make assumptions about their abilities or to talk over them. Instead, these experts advise speaking to the person directly, giving them time to respond, and not interrupting. It is usually helpful to minimize distractions; one-on-one communication in a quiet place often works well. In some cases it can also be beneficial to speak more slowly and to only ask one question at a time, to minimize the chance of misunderstanding or confusion.

As Alzheimer's progresses, many people find verbal communication more difficult and may need to use nonverbal methods like hand gestures as well. In their book *Six Steps to Managing Alzheimer's Disease and Dementia*, neurologist Andrew E. Budson and neuropsychologist Maureen K. O'Connor suggest using pictures to help with communication. They say, "If your loved one is having difficulty finding words or pronouncing them clearly, they may be able to point to a picture of what they want."[45] The authors also suggest looking for smartphone applications that are created for the purpose of picture-based communication. When it comes to communication, Alzheimer's experts also stress the importance of positivity—believing that communication and connection are possible—and coming up with creative ways to accomplish these goals.

Creative Ways to Connect

Experts also offer some creative ideas on activities that can be used to help connect with a person who has Alzheimer's. While everyone has unique likes and dislikes, many people report success with specific types of activities. One is to go outdoors or

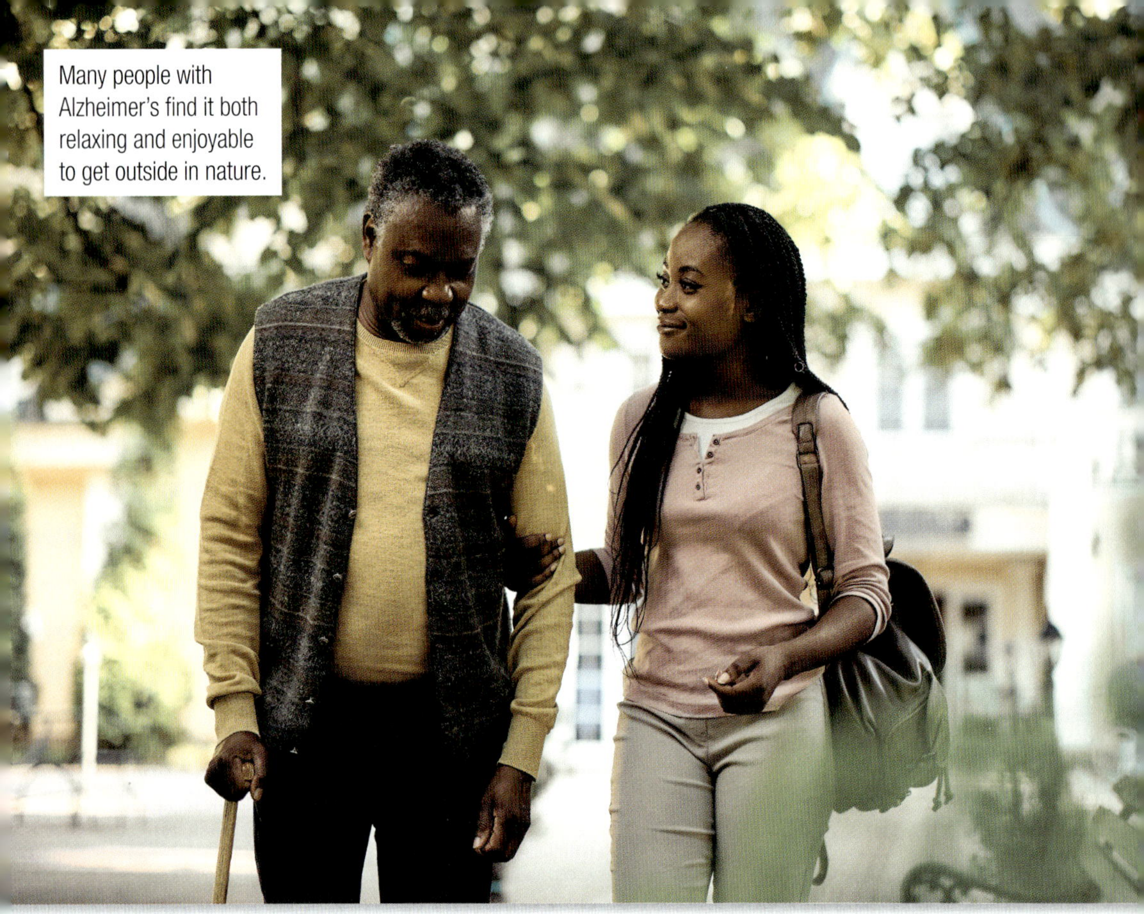

Many people with Alzheimer's find it both relaxing and enjoyable to get outside in nature.

have some type of contact with nature. Nature-related activities tend to be relatively simple and relaxing. One idea is to go for a walk (or if the person is in a wheelchair, take them for a walk), sit somewhere outside, or even find an inside spot with a view outside. Other ideas include gardening or getting an indoor plant, putting a bird feeder outside the window, or even getting a small pet like a fish or hamster. Barbara J. Huelat and Sharon T. Pochron, authors of *Taming the Chaos of Dementia*, explain that nature is an important part of human well-being. "Research shows that just sitting outside can have significant health benefits." One of the authors notes, "I've seen firsthand the positive impact that nature can have on people with dementia. My mom, who was no longer speaking, always wore a big smile when I took her on neighborhood wheelchair rides."[46]

"Research shows that just sitting outside can have significant health benefits."[46]

—Barbara J. Huelat and Sharon T. Pochron, authors of *Taming the Chaos of Dementia*

> "Try telling jokes together, looking at silly pictures of animals, watching a comedy, or anything that brings you both a smile."[48]
>
> —Gabrielle Stroubakis, dementia expert

Touch can be another effective way to connect. Physical contact can help people feel more relaxed and less anxious and is a great way to show love and compassion. Huelat and Pochron say, "Holding hands, giving a gentle shoulder touch, and hugging or kissing on the forehead can all communicate love and care. Manicures, pedicures, and other forms of personal care that involve gentle touch can also be beneficial."[47] However, while many people enjoy a gentle touch, it is important to always be mindful of another person's comfort and respond to their cues, since certain types of touch may also make someone feel uncomfortable.

While laughter might be one of the last things that comes to mind in relation to Alzheimer's, it can also be an effective way to connect. Writing for Alzheimer's San Diego, dementia expert Gabrielle Stroubakis explains that many aspects of communication change as Alzheimer's progresses, but "emotions remain a strong way to connect." She suggests, "Try telling jokes together, looking at silly pictures of animals, watching a comedy, or anything that brings you both a smile."[48]

Communication Can Be Unpredictable

Maureen Salamon, executive editor of *Harvard Women's Health Watch*, explains that one of the challenges in communicating with a person who has dementia is that every interaction can be different, meaning that it can be difficult to know what to expect and what strategies to use. She says, "A patient's ability to understand others and express themselves can fluctuate from day to day or even hour to hour." Suzanne Salamon, clinical chief of gerontology at Beth Israel Deaconess Medical Center, explains that this fluctuation is a result of what is happening in the brain. "If you think of the brain as millions of little electrical circuits with messages going from one area to another, a brain with dementia has areas that are clear and areas that are clogged up. Sometimes the electrical signals can find a clear path, and the person can answer more clearly; other times, messages get stuck. You don't know what you're going to get on any given day—and it's hard."

Maureen Salamon, "Bridging the Gap: Dementia Communication Strategies," Harvard Health, February 1, 2025. www.health.harvard.edu.

Interests and Memories That Are Often Preserved

Alzheimer's experts contend that while people with this disease may forget many things, certain types of memories are more likely to be preserved. Therefore, when trying to connect with someone with Alzheimer's, it can be helpful to tap into these memories. People with Alzheimer's typically have trouble remembering things that happened recently, so trying to have a conversation about what they did last week might not work. However, memories of the more distant past are stored in a different part of the brain and therefore are likely to remain intact for much longer. Health writer Stephanie Thurrott explains that not only are people with Alzheimer's more likely to remember things from the more distant past, but these memories can also be very comforting, and talking about them is likely to be enjoyable. She says, "Older memories are often nostalgic. They have emotional meaning. They may feel warm, familiar, secure and comfortable for people with Alzheimer's."[49] One way to access memories is to look at old photos, which can stimulate long-term memories and become starting points for conversations. Some people even create a small photo album that they can leave with their friend or family member who has Alzheimer's.

> "Often, people preserve their artistic abilities as they progress through their illness. Some even become a bit more creative."[50]
>
> —Carolyn Fredericks, Yale Medicine neurologist

Another type of memory that people with Alzheimer's tend to retain even when they forget many other things is their enjoyment of artistic activities. Yale Medicine neurologist Carolyn Fredericks says, "Often, people preserve their artistic abilities as they progress through their illness. Some even become a bit more creative."[50] She suggests using coloring books or arranging flowers as very simple artistic activities, or painting or sculpture as more complex options.

Music in particular is an artistic option that people with Alzheimer's tend to enjoy. They can often remember their favorite music even when they have forgotten many other things, and they find it enjoyable and calming to listen to familiar tunes. Leslie

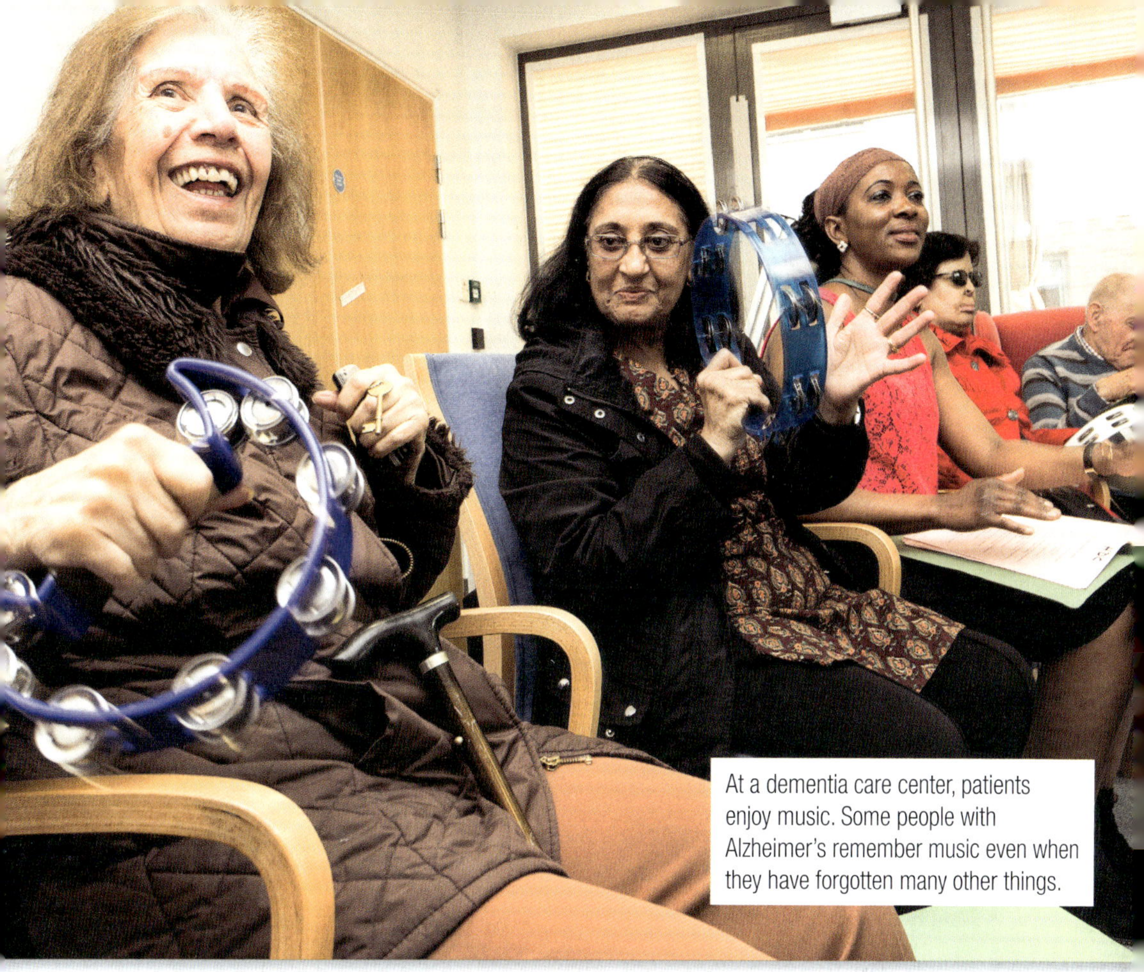

At a dementia care center, patients enjoy music. Some people with Alzheimer's remember music even when they have forgotten many other things.

Martin talks about how her father responds to music. She says, "Music really helps. My neighbor across the street is a jazz pianist, and I got him to come and play at the nursing home. Everybody was loving it. My dad hadn't talked for months and during one of the songs he started to cry. And when Arlington Jones, the jazz pianist, came over to say hello to us, my dad started talking to him."[51]

What Not to Do When Trying to Connect

To successfully connect, it is also important to understand what one should avoid doing. Certain types of actions can actually make connection more challenging. For instance, experts stress that it is not helpful to remind a person with Alzheimer's that they are forgetting things, because not only do they not have any control over this, but reminding them is likely to make them feel upset. Likewise, if someone is having trouble communicating, or if they start to get anxious or even angry when a conversation gets challenging, it is not beneficial to argue or get angry back at them, because this is likely to make the situation worse. As the authors of *Six Steps to Managing Alzheimer's Disease and Dementia*, explain, calm and gentle reassurance is usually a much better way to make the person feel comfortable and open up communication again. "Reassure them. Phrases like, 'You're safe,' 'Everything is OK,' and 'I'm here for you' can provide comfort."[52] In addition, they suggest that if connection becomes difficult, switching to a different approach or topic can be helpful. They explain, "When you redirect your loved one, you change the focus and direct them from the upsetting or counterproductive event or environment to something else."[53]

Is It Ever Okay to Lie?

A common question in relation to Alzheimer's is whether it is ever okay to lie to a person with this disease. As Alzheimer's progresses, a person might become confused about certain things, and telling them the truth might make them feel upset or agitated. On top of that, because memory problems are common with Alzheimer's, they might need to be told this same truth over and over again and as a result experience the same upset every time. An example of this is a person not remembering that a family member or other loved one has passed away. In a case like this, some people find that it is easier to lie because this is less emotionally distressing or less likely to provoke conflict. Matthew Domico and Valerie Hill, authors of *What You Need to Know About Alzheimer's Disease*, explain, "If the caregiver responds truthfully, the patient may experience a considerable grief reaction each time the question is asked, but by lying ('Mary is at the store'), caretakers can avoid such emotional upsets."[54]

Other people disagree with this position and argue that lying is never okay. They insist that lying damages the trust between

Alzheimer's and Reading

As Alzheimer's progresses and causes changes in memory and cognition, some people start to find that it is harder to enjoy their favorite activities. Experts stress that a person does not necessarily need to give up the activities they love but may just need to make some changes. For instance, many people love to read but start to find it challenging because they forget what they have read or cannot focus on a long novel. Yale Medicine neurologist Carolyn Fredericks suggests some ways to adapt rather than giving up reading altogether: "For some patients, what might work is finding shorter forms of reading. For one patient, she switched from reading books to magazines instead. For others, they could join a book club to benefit from the social aspect of it, which is more important than if they remember plot details."

Quoted in Carrie Macmillan, "How to Stay Connected with a Loved One with Alzheimer's Disease," Yale Medicine, January 30, 2024. www.yalemedicine.org.

two people, which can also damage a relationship. On its blog, North Point Living, which provides assisted living and memory care, offers some alternatives that allow caregivers to avoid upsetting people without having to lie. "A person with dementia might express worry about a deceased family member not coming home. Instead of saying, 'They're just out at the store,' you might reflect by responding, 'It sounds like you're missing them right now. Tell me more about what you loved doing together.' That validates their emotions without reinforcing the inaccurate belief." Another example is: "If an individual insists on going to work, a caregiver might redirect by saying, 'I see you're ready for a busy day. Before that, how about we go for a walk or look at some photos together?' This approach moves the focus away from the point of contention while respecting the person's sense of purpose."[55]

Meeting People Where They're At

The most effective approach to communication and connection will be different for everyone. In addition, even with a lot of forethought and the best intentions, connecting with a person who has Alzheimer's is likely to be difficult at times and might not go as planned. Some people who have dealt with the challenges of this disease conclude that one of the best approaches is to stop thinking about what has been lost, what is not working, and what they wish was different—even if only for a moment—and simply connect with the person who is in front of them at that moment. Owen Darnell, whose grandmother had Alzheimer's disease when Owen was a child, sums this philosophy up: "Alzheimer's disease taught me how to simply love people where they're at."[56]

Source Notes

Introduction: A Frighteningly Common Disease

1. Aidan Christy, "Exploring Dementia as I Remember My Grandmother," Mount St. Joseph University News, September 24, 2024. www.msj.edu.
2. Owen Darnell, "What Alzheimer's Disease Taught Me—a Narrative Dedicated to Mom," Senior Helping Seniors, May 17, 2019. https://shsboston.com.
3. Quoted in Alzheimer's Association, "What It's like Living with Alzheimer's," July 22, 2022. www.alz.org.

Chapter One: What Is Alzheimer's Disease?

4. Quoted in Reddit, "What Was Your Worse Senior Moment?," January 23, 2024. www.reddit.com.
5. Hailey Corum, "From Oatmeal Cookies to Soup on a Plate: An Alzheimer's Journey," Alzheimer's San Diego, 2025. www.alzsd.org.
6. Alzheimer's Association, "2025 Alzheimer's Disease Facts and Figures," 2025. www.alz.org.
7. Quoted in Emilie Le Beau Lucchesi, "A Personal Glimpse into Living with Symptoms of Early-Onset Alzheimer's," *Discover*, November 19, 2021. www.discovermagazine.com.
8. Quoted in Alzheimer's Association, "Alzheimer's: A Real Love Story . . . ," June 3, 2016. www.alz.org.
9. Emily Clionsky and Mitchell Clionsky, *Dementia Prevention: Using Your Head to Save Your Brain*. Johns Hopkins University Press, 2023, p. 18.
10. Jonathan Graff-Radford and Angela M. Lunde, *Mayo Clinic on Alzheimer's Disease and Other Dementias*. Mayo Clinic Press, 2025, p. 111.
11. Laury, "Laury's Story: 'Mum Became Utterly Lost in the Fog of Her Own Mind,'" Alzheimer's Society, September 20, 2019. www.alzheimers.org.uk.
12. Laury, "Laury's Story."
13. Centers for Disease Control and Prevention, "About Alzheimer's," August 15, 2024. www.cdc.gov.

Chapter Two: Why People Get Alzheimer's Disease

14. Quoted in Judith Graham, "Stalked by the Fear That Dementia Is Stalking You," KFF Health News, February 21, 2020. https://kffhealthnews.org.

15. Graff-Radford and Lunde, *Mayo Clinic on Alzheimer's Disease and Other Dementias*, p. 73.
16. Graff-Radford and Lunde, *Mayo Clinic on Alzheimer's Disease and Other Dementias*, p. 74.
17. National Institute on Aging, "Alzheimer's Disease Genetics Fact Sheet," March 1, 2023. www.nia.nih.gov.
18. Quoted in Laura Williamson, "Smoking Harms the Brain, Raises Dementia Risk—but Not If You Quit," American Heart Association, July 6, 2021. www.heart.org.
19. Alzheimer's Society, "Alcohol and the Risk of Dementia," 2025. www.alzheimers.org.uk.
20. Centers for Disease Control and Prevention, "Reducing Risk for Dementia," August 27, 2024. www.cdc.gov.
21. Donald Weaver, "Why Don't We Have a Cure for Alzheimer's Disease?," Alzheimer's Society, July 16, 2021. https://alzheimer.ca.

Chapter Three: How Alzheimer's Is Diagnosed and Treated

22. Quoted in UC Health, "Nancy's Story: Forging a New Path in Alzheimer's Treatment as UC Health's First Lecanemab Patient," December 11, 2023. www.uchealth.com.
23. Johns Hopkins Medicine, "Alzheimer's Disease Overview," 2025. www.hopkinsmedicine.org.
24. Graff-Radford and Lunde, *Mayo Clinic on Alzheimer's Disease and Other Dementias*, p. 97.
25. Quoted in Alzheimer's Research UK, "How Larry's Experience on New Treatment for Alzheimer's Offers Hope for Future," September 17, 2025. www.alzheimersresearchuk.org.
26. Graff-Radford and Lunde, *Mayo Clinic on Alzheimer's Disease and Other Dementias*, p. 130.
27. Alzheimer's Association, "Treatments for Behavior," 2025. www.alz.org.
28. Quoted in Alzheimer Scotland, "Willy's Story," 2025. www.alzscot.org.
29. Lisa Catanese, "Memory Care: A Senior Living Option for Those with Dementia or Alzheimer's Disease," Harvard Health, October 9, 2024. www.health.harvard.edu.
30. Quoted in Madeline North, "8 Recent Breakthroughs in the Fight Against Alzheimer's Disease," World Economic Forum, June 27, 2025. www.weforum.org.

31. Quoted in Alzheimer's Research UK, "'We're Moving into a Completely Different World. Treatments for Dementia Are Coming,'" December 19, 2024. www.alzheimersresearchuk.org.

Chapter Four: How Alzheimer's Disease Affects People and Their Families

32. Quoted in Alzheimer's New Jersey, "Janice's Alzheimer's Story," September 5, 2024. www.alznj.org.
33. Rick Phelps, "What It Really Feels like to Have Alzheimer's Disease," AgingCare, 2025. www.agingcare.com.
34. Peter, "Peter's Story: 'I Don't Worry About the Things I Can't Do—There's No Point Struggling,'" Dementia UK, 2025. www.dementiauk.org.
35. Cheryl Liddell, comment on Alzheimer's Society post, Facebook, July 25, 2025. www.facebook.com.
36. Katie Stevens, "The Hardest Goodbye: A Granddaughter's Story,' Alzheimer's Association, October 21, 2016. www.alz.org.
37. Lizzie Thomson, "This Is How It Feels to Watch a Loved One Suffer with Alzheimer's," The Tab, May 15, 2016. https://archive.thetab.com.
38. Quoted in Lindsay Clein, "'It's Hard to Watch Somebody Just Disappear:' Triad Woman Shares Touching Story of Husband's Alzheimer's Battle," WXII12, June 20, 2025. www.wxii12.com.
39. Quoted in Darlene Donloe, "Alzheimer's Caregivers Share Stories of Stress, Heartache," Center for Health Journalism, September 16, 2021. https://centerforhealthjournalism.org.
40. Cameron Huddleston, "What It's Really like When Your Parent Has Alzheimer's Disease," Cameron Huddleston personal website, September 10, 2020. https://cameronhuddleston.com.
41. Alzheimer's Society of Canada, "What Does Stigma Against Dementia Look Like?," 2025. https://alzheimer.ca.
42. Quoted in Peter Reed et al., "Transcending the Tragedy Discourse of Dementia: An Ethical Imperative for Promoting Selfhood, Meaningful Relationships, and Well-Being," *AMA Journal of Ethics*, July 2017. https://journalofethics.ama-assn.org.
43. Lindsey Ko, "Alzheimer's Disease: A Teenager's Perspective," Alzheimer's Orange County, 2025. www.alzoc.org.

Chapter Five: Ways to Connect with People Who Have Alzheimer's

44. Limensor, "My Grandma," Reddit, June 13, 2022. www.reddit.com.
45. Andrew E. Budson and Maureen K. O'Connor, *Six Steps to Managing Alzheimer's Disease and Dementia: A Guide for Families*. Oxford University Press, 2022, p. 80.
46. Barbara J. Huelat and Sharon T. Pochron, *Taming the Chaos of Dementia: A Caregiver's Guide to Interventions That Make a Difference*. Rowman & Littlefield, 2023, p. 153.
47. Huelat and Pochron, *Taming the Chaos of Dementia*, p. 179.
48. Gabrielle Stroubakis, "Using Humor Throughout the Dementia Journey," Alzheimer's San Diego, 2025. www.alzsd.org.
49. Stephanie Thurrott, "Why People with Alzheimer's Disease Might Live in the Past," Banner Health, April 17, 2024. www.bannerhealth.com.
50. Quoted in Carrie Macmillan, "How to Stay Connected with a Loved One with Alzheimer's Disease," Yale Medicine, January 30, 2024. www.yalemedicine.org.
51. Quoted in Mind Crowd, "Alzheimer's Stories: Interview with Leslie Martin, Author of 'Forgotten Tomorrows, Crazy Todays,'" 2025. https://mindcrowd.org.
52. Andrew E. Budson and Maureen K. O'Connor, *Six Steps to Managing Alzheimer's Disease and Dementia: A Guide for Families*, pp. 39–40.
53. Budson and O'Connor, *Six Steps to Managing Alzheimer's Disease and Dementia*, p. 41.
54. Matthew Domico and Valerie Hil, *What You Need to Know About Alzheimer's Disease*. Greenwood, 2022, p. 112.
55. North Point Living, "Is Lying to a Person with Dementia Ethical?," April 30, 2023. www.pegasusseniorliving.com.
56. Owen Darnell, "What Alzheimer's Disease Taught Me—a Narrative Dedicated to Mom."

For Further Research

Books

Andrew E. Budson and Maureen K. O'Connor, *Six Steps to Managing Alzheimer's Disease and Dementia: A Guide for Families*. Oxford University Press, 2022.

Emily Clionsky and Mitchell Clionsky, *Dementia Prevention: Using Your Head to Save Your Brain*. Johns Hopkins University Press, 2023.

Jonathan Graff-Radford and Angela M. Lunde, *Mayo Clinic on Alzheimer's Disease and Other Dementias*. Mayo Clinic Press, 2025.

Barbara J. Huelat and Sharon T. Pochron, *Taming the Chaos of Dementia: A Caregiver's Guide to Interventions That Make a Difference*. Rowman & Littlefield, 2023.

Internet Sources

Alzheimer's Association, "2025 Alzheimer's Disease Facts and Figures," 2025. www.alz.org.

Centers for Disease Control and Prevention, "About Alzheimer's," August 15, 2024. www.cdc.gov.

Johns Hopkins Medicine, "Alzheimer's Disease Overview," 2025. www.hopkinsmedicine.org.

National Institute on Aging, "How Is Alzheimer's Treated?," September 12, 2023. www.nia.nih.gov.

Madeline North, "8 Recent Breakthroughs in the Fight Against Alzheimer's Disease," World Economic Forum, June 27, 2025. www.weforum.org.

Organizations and Websites

Alzheimer's Association

www.alz.org

The Alzheimer's Association is a nonprofit organization that works to accelerate research, improve treatments, and ultimately end Alzheimer's. Its website has information about the symptoms of this disease, its stages, how it is diagnosed, treatments, and research. It publishes the yearly *Alzheimer's Disease Facts and Figures* report.

Alzheimer's Foundation of America
https://alzfdn.org
This organization provides support and education for people affected by Alzheimer's. Its website contains a variety of educational resources, including facts about the disease, information about what to do after diagnosis, and information about the early-onset form of Alzheimer's.

Alzheimers.gov
www.alzheimers.gov
Alzheimers.gov is the federal government website that links users to a wide variety of information about Alzheimer's, for the purpose of support and education. It is managed by the National Institutes of Health and includes information about what it is like to have Alzheimer's, tips for caregivers, and information about clinical trials.

Alzheimer's Society
www.alzheimers.org.uk
This organization is based in the United Kingdom and is devoted to better understanding Alzheimer's and supporting the people affected by it. Its website has information about what Alzheimer's is, how it is diagnosed and treated, and how to reduce risk. There are also numerous personal stories related to living with the disease.

National Institute on Aging (NIA)
www.nia.nih.gov
The NIA is part of the National Institutes of Health and works to better understand and improve the aging process. It conducts research on Alzheimer's, and its website has information about the causes and risk factors of the disease, as well as about diagnosis, treatment, and caregiving.

Index

Picture Credits

Cover: PeopleImages/Shutterstock

6: Ocskay Mark/Shutterstock
9: Dmytro Zinkevych/Shutterstock
12: Kotcha K/Shutterstock
15: Photodjo/iStock
18: Science History Images/Alamy Images
19: Science History Images/Alamy Images
23: halfpoint/Shutterstock
28: Gorodenkoff/Shutterstock
30: kmpzzz/Shutterstock
32: Toa55/Shutterstock
38: Krakenimages.com/Shutterstock
41: JU.STOCKER/Shutterstock
43: SB Arts Media/Shutterstock
46: Monkey Business Images/Shutterstock
48: Drazen Zigic/Shutterstock
51: John Birdsall/Alamy Images

About the Author

Andrea C. Nakaya holds a bachelor of arts in English and a master of arts in communications from San Diego State University. She has written and edited hundreds of articles and more than fifty books on current issues. She currently lives in Eagle, Idaho.